THE CODE OF THE MASTERS

THE CODE OF THE MASTERS
UNIVERSAL KABBALAH WITH NAAM YOGA

DR. JOSEPH MICHAEL LEVRY

⊙ **Root**light, Inc.
NEW YORK, NY

Also by Dr. Joseph Michael Levry:
Alchemy of Love Relationships
Lifting the Veil: The Divine Code
The Divine Doctor: Healing Beyond Medicine
The Healing Fire of Heaven

Copyright ©2006 Joseph Michael Levry. Revised 2007.

Rootlight, Inc. 15 Park Avenue, Suite 7C New York, NY 10016
www.rootlight.com

All rights reserved. This book is protected under the copyright laws of the United States of America. This book may not be copied or reprinted for commercial gain or profit. This book may not be reproduced in whole or in part, or by any means electronic, mechanical, photocopying, recording, or other, without express written permission from the publisher, except by a reviewer who may use brief passages in a review.

DESIGN: *Renée R. Skuba*
PHOTOGRAPHY: *Marni Lustig* and *Jesus Mico*
MODELS: *Alyssa Gaustad* and *Renata Spironello*

Printed in the United States of America
For Worldwide Distribution
ISBN 978-1-885562-25-8

Printed on recycled paper

CONTENTS

Foreword vii
Introduction 1
Chapter 1: The Hidden Forces in Our Hands 29
Chapter 2: Naam Yoga and Universal Kabbalah 61
   Meditation for Attracting the Energy of Jupiter 79
   Meditation for Maturity and Wisdom 80
   Harmonize the Brain for Maximum Effectiveness 81
Chapter 3: Divine Spiritual Wisdom 83
Chapter 4: The Fall of Man 97
Chapter 5: The Pattern of Creation: 3–7–12 103
Chapter 6: The Nature of Man 113
   Meditation: Sodarchan Chakra Kriya 119
Chapter 7: The Age of the Christos 121
Chapter 8: The Star of Great Light 137
Chapter 9: Truth 145
Chapter 10: I Am That I Am 149
Chapter 11: Children 155
   Meditation: I Am, I Am 159
Chapter 12: The Way of the Heart 163
   Meditation to Connect with Your Heart 171
Chapter 13: The Heart Center 173
   Meditation to Brighten Your Radiance 178
Chapter 14: The Way of Service 179
Chapter 15: The Seven Archangels 189
Chapter 16: Our Planetary Bodies 199
   Tenth Body Meditation 202
Chapter 17: The Power of Sacred Music 203
Chapter 18: Lumen de Lumine 209
   Meditation for Bringing in Light 213
Chapter 19: Achieving Cosmic Consciousness 217
   Meditation to Awaken Your Highest Destiny 227
Chapter 20: The Healing Spirit of Ra Ma Da Sa 229
   The Lion's Heart Series 238
Chapter 21: The Bones 253
Chapter 22: Harmonyum: The Unknown Medicine 259
Chapter 23: The Splendor of Naam Yoga 265
Conclusion 269

*Naam is the crown of sacred wisdom.
It enhances the development of the
dormant faculty within us that allows us
to perceive hidden, eternal truths.
The opening of this spiritual faculty
represents the mystery of regeneration—
the vital union between God and man.*

FOREWORD

A TRUE SPIRITUAL MASTER

Reading this work with an open heart will bring light to your mind, peace to your heart and strength to your spirit. Before I begin, I need to acknowledge the Rose Croix Kabbalah Initiates and Masters who guided me at an early age and imparted this once secret and vast Divine Spiritual Science to me; for from Divine Spiritual Wisdom emanates all wisdom, all knowledge and all guidance. I am extremely grateful to the late Master of White Tantric and Kundalini Yoga, Yogi Bhajan, the Siri Singh Sahib, who lovingly supported me throughout the many years, and encouraged me to merge the holy Kabbalah with Kundalini Yoga. For it is he who said, "It took me (Yogi Bhajan) 40 years to learn this science and it took you (Joseph Michael Levry) to write it down. This work shall live forever." I am also deeply grateful to Maharaj Ji for giving me the Naam while I was in India. Babaji is a holy person of biblical proportions whose powerful spirituality was first recognized when he was a child. It was Baba Siri Chand Ji, the great sixteenth-century yogi, mystic and elder son of Guru Nanak Dev Ji, the first Sikh Guru, who appeared to him and instructed him. Not long thereafter, Baba Siri Chand Ji returned with his father Guru Nanak Dev Ji. Guru Nanak gave him the Naam. As a boy, Babaji began healing intractable diseases, bringing the dead back to life and transforming people's lives. Villagers soon recognized that great spiritual powers were developing within him. Maharaj Ji is a true symbol of holiness, humility and service.

The Master helps the student reach his/her highest destiny and find the real Master within. Indeed, the real Master, the God of your heart, is always living in you, in your heart. This is the One Truth.

One of the highest blessings that you can receive from God while living on earth is to meet a True Spiritual Master. It is like finding your second mother, for a Master is the One through whom you will be born into the higher world. A True Spiritual Master is the Word Made Flesh. Finding one is a precious treasure, for a Master is the incarnation of the Word, or Naam. A True Master will teach you the exact divine science, the exact spiritual technology, the exact celestial knowledge which will allow you to connect with and experience the highest, purest wisdom in this universe. He will transmit to you the nourishing fire that gives the strength to act upon everything in nature. He will give you the golden key that opens the gate of mystery. By working with a True Master, a person can experience direct connection with the Spirit of God, and the unseen realm, so that one may receive unimaginable celestial treasures and the spiritual knowledge of all natural things.

The True Master will show you how to work with the forces of nature, planetary powers and zodiacal stars to heal yourself and serve others. He will reveal to you the secret of the inner Kabbalah along with the highest form of yoga. By working with a True Master, you can receive the graceful method of awakening Cosmic Consciousness, so that you experience an unusual joy which no one can take away. Working under a True Master is the beginning of the manifestation of the human soul. He will cause your soul to rise and display its timeless beauty. A True Master will open your heart so that Divine warmth can flow into it, and you may experience Divine joy and gladness. He will help you see the light of your soul, which will cast its beam far and wide, enabling you to see the indescribable wonder of God, nature and Man. God gives the Master, and the Master gives you God through the science of Naam. In this life there are two great gifts: the first is prana, the breath of life, and the second is a spiritual teacher or Master. Both gifts are given by the Grace of God. A True Master, then, is the pure vehicle through which the soul can connect with God.

A True Master will be known by his vast and magnetic aura that looks like the sun, and by his simple, direct and down-to-earth way. His words touch the heart because they emanate from one who serves thousands of lives as the conduit of the Divine energy. He is the Word Made Flesh, and the heavenly force is transmitted through his very presence. The aura and blessings of a True Spiritual Master can bring the entire psyche and being of those in his presence into balance. In the play of human existence, the True Spiritual Master is a different sort of being. His life is only sacrifice and, therefore, it contains more problems to resolve than that of the ordinary soul. His life is never his own, as he sacrifices his personal comforts in order to serve and transmute the karma of all with whom he comes into contact. The more the Master yields to his Divine function, however, the more powers become available to him. While he is the sacrificial embodiment of Divine Consciousness, the Master is still subject to some of the limitations of human existence. During his lifetime, he is transfigured and awakened to his Divine purpose. The life of a Master is one of constant service and communication of the Divine Spiritual Wisdom that is passed down through the ages.

A True Spiritual Master understands the pains of the world, as well as how to access the channels of cosmic energy in order to mitigate those pains. The majority of people are held captive by their destructive patterns caused by the seven negative karmic influences. It is only through Naam, and the help and guidance of a True Spiritual Master, that these people can be assisted in overcoming their bad habits. A True Spiritual Master will teach you that nothing occurs by chance, and nothing is based on probability. Everything on your life's journey is directly related to your focus on self-improvement and your spiritual practice. Some of the hardships you experience are the obstacles you have created through the karma that you've accrued. Yet, karma can become a blessing. No matter how tumultuous a time you have been through, or how much more is required, you can't be attached to time. In general, eliminating all karma for a student is not permitted, and while a Master can help, every student must repay their karma. After the karmic arrangements are made prior to re-entering the realm of the earth, nothing other than Naam, along with the guidance of a True Spiritual Master, can change your karmic debt. To do otherwise would be to violate the Laws of Heaven.

If you do Naam to merge with God, your illness will be healed. If you do Naam for the purpose of healing your illness, then the illness will not be healed. It is only by merging with God, which is Naam, that the goal will be achieved. Human bodies are meant to repay karma, and some karma manifests as illness. Therefore, practice Naam, receive Harmonyum Healing and give up your attachment to healing your illnesses. As a matter of fact, the Harmonyum Healing System will help you give up your attachments so that you may create the platform for self-healing. Interestingly, when you do Naam Yoga, you are spared collective karma, though you still have to deal with your individual karma. When a person is going through cycles of reincarnation in the human realm, he is reincarnating in the midst of hardship no matter how great his life is, and no matter how blessed he may be. For Naam Yogis, everything you owed in the past will be repaid and settled through the bestowal of blessings upon you through Naam. Also, the tribulations that you experience while going through your spiritual practice are meant to pay for the karmic debts that you owe. Even though the increased hardship might render you unable to practice, you should still endeavor to keep up with your work.

When a Naam Yogi is about to run into trouble, the energy force of the Naam will dissolve the obstacles on his/her path. Naam can also give you signs and warnings of events to come. When you are dedicated to the sacred wisdom passed on to you by a Master who truly works with the unseen world, some angels may appear in your dreams or before your eyes to share things with you. If your level of spiritual evolution is not high enough, they will not let you see them, but they can let you know through signs. There are times when these luminous beings will let you see them in your sleep, often when you are in a dream state. Certain people can see luminous beings consistently in their dreams. If your ability to concentrate is very good, you may also see these helpful beings during meditation. However, if you desire to see them only for the pleasure of doing so, meaning that your desire to see them is motivated by your ego, you will not be allowed to see them. As long as you practice Divine Spiritual Wisdom for the purpose of merging with God, you will surely be able to see these luminous beings in the future.

Healing an average person takes his/her whole life and entails balancing his/her karmic relationships simultaneously in various dimensions. All those debts must be resolved benevolently in order for the ailments of this lifetime to be resolved. Some people accumulate a lot of karma. People leave this life with both the white light they have gained through doing service and good deeds, along with the black light from the negative karma they have collected. Normally, the elimination of karma cannot be done unconditionally, nor can it all be eliminated for you. It is said in the sacred teachings that you cannot succeed in seeing the unseen in one lifetime, and that only after a few reincarnations can you succeed in accomplishing this task. Basically, you are unable to eliminate that much karma all at once. Your capacity to see the unseen is proportional to how much karma you resolve.

A True Spiritual Master understands that each student must venture into the positive and negative side of things in order to wash out their karmic garbage and cleanse their psyches of that which has been holding them down for many lifetimes. It takes time, energy and patience on the part of a True Master to polish the rough edges of each student so that he/she is able to effectively communicate the teachings. You can pack a donkey with many holy books, but it will never be a priest. Therefore, it takes a tremendous amount of willingness on the part of the student; willingness to do the hard work necessary for authentic transformation. Initially, when the Master begins to polish the stone, the stone cries out, "Why does he chisel me?" But, after a time, as the stone becomes precious, it recognizes how necessary the chisel was, how vital it was to polish. As a result, you leave your old life and enter into the new one with a new understanding. When working with a True Master, he will both help you, and get on your case. This will make you strong enough to handle the pressure that comes with being out in the world on your own. It is a great privilege when the Master is harsh on you, because Gold is known by the fire it goes through. Remember, all Masters were once students who were also taken through the fire by their Masters. All must pass through the same door in order to become strong. It cannot be otherwise. The most difficult thing to do is win the heart of a True Master. When you do so, you are winning the heart of the Cosmic Mother. Thousands of people come before the True Spiritual Master. Through a screening process, he chooses to work with those who are truly devotional. And, among the devotional, he screens again to find the most devotional one. In essence, the student is the baby to the Master. As such, the student is secure when he/she is holding onto the mother with all his/her might. The relationship that develops between the Master and the student is a healing, Divine bond. Nobody can break it. Through this relationship, the Master helps the student reach his/her highest destiny and find the real Master within. Indeed, the real Master, the God of your heart, is always living in you, in your heart. This is the One Truth.

When a Master takes you under his wing, it is a privilege and a blessing. Those who serve a Master do so unconditionally and with love in their hearts. They are set on a path of mastery themselves, committed to serving all others. In fact, in serving the Master, you are also serving the thousands of beings that he serves, creating a chain of humility in the name of the Divine. Sacrifice will come naturally to you, as you will be returning a portion of the profound gifts you have received. Gratitude will fill your heart for the miracles of your life and wonder for the miracles in the lives of those around you. Even if you experience a tangle of complications that seem irresolvable, the light of the Divine will resolve them at the last minute – always in the very nick of time. Gratitude becomes a natural part of your life, especially to the one who has liberated you and shown you the Power of the Word and continues to direct your life in the path of that heavenly Light. Once you find a True Master and surrender to God, Naam, and your path, do not turn back. Completely surrender to the Divine Spiritual Wisdom and dedicate your life to Naam. That is pure dedication. You will win and reach your highest, loftiest achievement. By treating a True Spiritual Master with reverence, we are awakened to our ultimate destiny and the God-realizing process of existence, and Heaven comes through in all realms of our lives.

The fastest way to grow spiritually and see the unseen, is to take the bull by the horns and open your heart to the Master. The Master doesn't care whether you are good or bad. For him, everything is always good.

The Master will always teach you to live in the positive, and die in the positive. That is the higher way of life. Walk one step toward the Master with a pure heart, and the Master will walk two steps toward you. The Master teaches you how to serve so that you may awaken those forces through which the negative karmic ties of the past can be eradicated, so that you may enter into a life of freedom. He will teach you that service is the way to heal all ills. When faced with mental, emotional and/or physical challenges, learn the Divine Spiritual Wisdom, vibrate Naam, serve others and serve God. This will cause your problems to vanish. Those who vibrate Naam and serve God are given the favorable conditions they need to blossom and be happy. They do not need to be concerned with what may occur because in the end, regardless of what happens, miracles will bless their lives. These people are protected by the elements of ether, air, fire, water and earth. They are able to receive the beneficial healing forces emitted by the cosmos. Serving others is a meditation in and of itself, and the highest form of yoga.

When the heavens arrange for you to meet the Master, it is your specific destiny, for you cannot override the heavens. Your entire life will be transformed, and your spiritual, emotional and mental growth will be exponential. You may even feel at times as if you are flying through waves of knowledge, sensing that all is changing around you. The light of the Master, who is one of the generations of the Universal Repairer, touches you, working through you to improve the lives of all around you, so you, too, become the conduit of the heavens. Your relationship with yourself will change as you become brighter, clearer, more focused and capable of others' trust in you. You will become the living Word as its divinity comes to live in you. Then, your relationship with your family will change. As you work on yourself via the heavenly light, this light will benefit your family and smooth the paths of discord. This will extend to your relationships with all beings, creating a ripple effect – a wave of light that passes from one person to the next.

When you give to a Master, you automatically receive blessings. The Master is constantly sowing seeds of Goodness by turning thousands of people to the Light of God. He is opening thousands of hearts to God, with his words, his touch, his presence, his deeds and his works. He gives and serves thousands of people. The Master serves on a daily basis those who are in dire need and helps those overcome with sorrow, pain and sickness. God serves the True Spiritual Master because he serves others as an extension of God. By giving to a Master, you give, through him, to the thousands of people he serves. By giving to the True Spiritual Master you will receive blessings from the thousands of people you have served through him. In your time of need, the universe will automatically provide for you. Giving to a True Spiritual Master opens the channels to Divine Good within and without. It opens in our consciousness the way for spiritual growth and supply to come to us. It brings us in direct contact with spiritual life, substance and intelligence. It loosens the burdens of our personal lives, unifies us with the universe and opens within and without an inflow and outflow of God's bounty.

When you leave this world, all the material richness that you may have acquired in this life is left behind. However, every good deed that you have done will go with you. Those who have served in this life will attract material and spiritual richness in their next life. Abundance follows the Law of Service. When the student serves the Master unconditionally, he/she is automatically on the path of becoming a Master in this, or another, lifetime. Then the student is able to help many, many people as well. In so doing, the student receives untold happiness. Indeed, as others benefit from what the student is now able to give, his/her soul rises higher and higher, becoming increasingly powerful and bright like the Sun. Meeting a True Master, then, is a precious gift; a chance to move from fate to destiny.

When one decides to work under a True Spiritual Master, he blesses you with the Naam and helps you free yourself of the burden of fate, so that you may manifest your highest destiny. It is vital to "Know thyself, to learn to die before death." To know the method of dying before death we need a True Master who has experienced such a death. He will bless you with Naam, and teach the method of dying before death. A man must learn to die once, so that he may not want to die again. When dying, one loses the desire to eat. Then the desire to breathe is progressively cut off, causing you to breathe less air. As a result, one learns to eat with love and to breathe with love. God created man to eat with love, think with love, feel with love, speak with love and to act with love. This sacred fire must be the reason that stimulates man. It is not an easy thing for a person to learn without a Master, for he can teach you how to take care of your blood, in which the spiritual alchemy must take place. The Master instructs you on how to purify your blood so that the Holy Spirit may incarnate in you. You cannot purify your blood if you do not have pure thoughts, pure feelings, pure speech and pure actions. When you study with a Master, you learn the Law of Purification so that even your blood may become purified. When you purify your blood you will get rid of thousands of diseases that derive from impurities in the bloodstream. A true Master teaches you how to eat pure and clean food, and shows you the right way to drink hot water so that you may remove thousands of diseases due to impure food and keep them at bay. Unclean and impure food brings filth into your stomach, which fouls the blood years later and inspires pessimism and poor health overall. A person with pure blood is always lively. If you lose your liveliness, your blood is impure. A Master can show you how the cultivation of pure thought, pure feelings, and pure actions result in pure blood, lively spirits, and abundant health and youth.

Working with a True Spiritual Master will cause you to go through a process of regeneration in which there will be a sublimation of vice into virtue. You will be reborn in the Spirit whereby the body and soul are penetrated by the heat of Divine Love and the light of Divine Intelligence that emanates from the Divine Fire held within self-consciousness and self-knowledge. The True Master will help you develop the Heavenly Rose, also known as the lost inner faculty, so that you may perceive the hidden, eternal truths. The opening of this spiritual faculty and blossoming of the Heavenly Rose is the mystery of regeneration – the vital union between God and Man. Human beings in the modern world are living in exile, deprived of their true essence and real powers.

We are creatures of opposites, a battleground for good and evil that consists of the imperishable, metaphysical substance and the material, perishable substance that fight within us. The imperishable remains enclosed in the perishable; in other words, within our mortal shells exist a mighty spiritual body. We need a True Spiritual Master to learn the true method of regeneration, in order to loosen the corruptible matter that keeps our immortal being bound in chains, and the active power asleep. It is the inner spiritual organ that has an incorruptible, transcendental, metaphysical essence as its foundation. All our misery springs from our corruptible material of mortality. For Man to be freed from this misery, it is necessary for the immortal, incorruptible principle residing within our inner being to be developed so that it is able, as it were, to devour the corruptible and the mortal. We must experience a rebirth in which the spirit of wisdom and love rules and the animal nature obeys, establishing the conditions whereby we are able to enter into communication with the world of higher intelligences. To this end, we need a True Master, who will show us, while in the human form, how the Soul can realize God and retrace its footsteps to reach its first home. This Divine Spiritual Wisdom brings joy and expansion. The teachings of the Masters will lead you to self-realization and Cosmic Consciousness through an all-embracing love and selfless service of humankind. Those who are truly intrigued are automatically led to the right place by the Light of God within them. Those who have a strong desire for Divine Spiritual Wisdom can receive guidance from a True Master long before they come into the physical presence of the Master – the one who represents the Word Made Flesh.

In this life, it is important to find a true living Master who is able to impart to you, through Naam, the everlasting inner connection of the soul with God, and who will guide you until you reach the goal of oneness with God. The Master appears when the student is ready. Once found, your Spiritual Master will teach you the Divine Spiritual Wisdom and initiate you with the science of Naam. Upon initiation into the vast heavenly science, you are then charged with maintaining a connection with the three Circles of Light. The first Circle of Light corresponds to the physical plane, and is activated by your pure love for the Master. The second Circle of Light corresponds to the astral plane, and is activated by your love for the teachings. The third Circle of Light corresponds to the divine plane, and is activated by your love of God. It is very rare to encounter a living Master who works with the unseen. When a Master can perceive the unseen, he is possessed of a pure and massive desire to serve mankind and has only been given this knowledge in order to further his service. When you merge with such a Master, he gives you a taste of the unseen by teaching you the various laws of nature that govern life. Then all your inner faculties will begin to open, and you will understand things as you have never understood them before. Your heart will be purified, and you will communicate from an open, loving stance that is nourished and fortified by the Living Word that the True Master embodies. Time and space do not interfere with the work of a Master. The Power of the Master is all-pervading and not confined to any one place.

The gifts of a Master are priceless. Only the currency of this Divine Spiritual Wisdom given to you by a Master allows you to navigate through this world and the higher dimensions. Understand that sex, money and power will never go past your last breath. It is the Divine Spiritual Wisdom you have learned and all the good that you have done while living on the earth that will remain with you and follow you into the hereafter. Divine Spiritual Wisdom is the only currency used in all the other dimensions beyond the earth. The fact is, no amount of money can buy you a car or a house in the higher world. It just doesn't work that way. Authentic spiritual wealth causes the universe to take care of you in this lifetime and beyond. Also, the words and advice of a True Master will always be effective and in the highest interest of the student, and will always produce results. When you read the work of a Master, no matter where you are, the power of his words subtly and distinctively penetrate to the core of your being and begin changing you. A real Master will not interfere with your fate or your free will, but will guide you gracefully. You alone will change to the measure in which you are ready, as the heavenly light always gives you free will. You will develop psychic spiritual powers, becoming one of the thousand hands of Heaven that love to serve and bring great joy to the world.

Humankind usually lives in a degraded state, however, the path of Naam will give you the highest spiritual strength and true grace. It is important to keep in mind that no yoga posture can open the heart; only Naam can do it. Work to serve the soul, and through humility and selfless service you will achieve true happiness. The crown of sacred wisdom, which is Naam, gracefully and sweetly arouses the dormant power within and makes a person all-knowing, peaceful and full of light. When we vibrate the Naam, we expand the breath and contract through the heart, which causes us to digest heavenly light. By focusing on the third eye or seat of the soul, and vibrating Naam, we are lifted and carried up by the sound current from one plane to the other until we become All-knowing, All-pervading and All-powerful, embracing the totality of His being.

Naam makes one as perfect as is the Father in Heaven. Besides physical health, it bestows mental and spiritual equilibrium, which is the health of spirit and on which the health of both the body and the mind depends. The spiritual journey starts by going within because this is the true pathway toward the kingdom of God. By rising above the physical body, one grows in awareness and consciousness of a higher order. Vibrating Naam lifts the soul beyond time and space. Naam is the heavenly food of the most perfect and God-like beings, a celestial diet that gives us radiant health and the nourishment to fulfill our destiny. Naam enhances the development of the dormant faculty within us that allows us to perceive hidden, eternal truths. The opening of this spiritual faculty represents the mystery of regeneration – the vital union between God and man. Readiness is achieved by developing the willingness to serve your fellow man. Humility and service are the keys that enable us to open the door.

The Master takes you in and guides you upward because the way of Naam lies inward and upward. By vibrating Naam we knock on the door of Heaven, so that it may be opened to us. It is especially important to repeat Naam without disturbing the steady and intently penetrating gaze emanating from the All-seeing eye; the third eye. With Naam you will be taken into the upper world where you will experience things neither seen nor heard, nor ever conceived of before. Ascending from one spiritual plane to another gives greater awakening and an awareness of a higher level. Naam allows us to ascend from the physical to the astral planes, and then to the divine plane.

To those of you on the path of light and service, who are being faced with gossip and criticism, just keep in mind that if all the criticism and resistance represented by the forces of darkness were eliminated from our lives, the power of goodness would be left unmanifest and by the lack of comparison would remain unqualified and perhaps unknown. If there were no such thing in the electric circuit as a small globe containing a wire of high resistance, the electric current flowing through the wires in our homes and offices would never produce any light to dispel the darkness. The resistance offered by the fine wire acts as a challenge to the flow of electric energy, the same force that attempts to stop it, curtail it, to checkmate its rhythmic surge, is what produces in the electric globe, a light.

There are always challenges in spreading the Work of Light, but these obstacles inspire the greater light to be revealed. Nothing can destroy a servant of the universe from carrying out the Work of Light and serving others. They are protected by the higher worlds, the Lord of the invisible Community of Light. There is a Cosmic law which states that regardless of how seriously, how costly, and how sadly a servant of light is forced to labor as a result of the unpleasant, unkind, and incorrect activities of the representatives of the darker forces, and regardless of how greatly he/she personally suffers in time, effort, and mental concern, it will always be known to them that they are protected by the Light of Heaven, and must carry on without one degree of concession to the fictitious claims and attitudes of these unevolved beings and representatives of the forces of darkness. When people criticize and gossip about you they are doing you a big favor. It's the best PR you can find. Cook these obstacles with the fire of Naam and transform them into your breakfast.

A Spiritual Master is not disturbed by opposites. He will teach you that everything in this world is perishable, and the only constant is change. He will show you that in order to find permanent peace in this unstable world, we must find Naam. Naam does not die. Therefore, by uniting ourselves with the Word, we are released from the cycle of re-birth and find our seat in the home of God where there is eternal peace. Understand that in order to find peace and happiness on this earth, we must unite our soul with God through Naam. This is the only union that will make us truly happy. A True Spiritual Master who is already united with God can impart the method of uniting with God through Naam, for a true living Master is one who has been commissioned by God to reconnect souls. The crown of a True Spiritual Master is only bestowed by the heavens.

The Wisdom and Teachings of a Master will confirm and bring into perspective all that you have previously discovered and practiced. It is then up to you to maintain the rigorous adherence to truth and selflessness required to reach the highest summits of the spirit. The Master neither reacts nor judges. He will only act in harmony with the heavens, and he will teach you that succumbing to reactions only creates additional karma. He will show you how to enter the eye of the storm so that you may escape the turbulent, destructive power of karma. He will lovingly teach you that all situations must be faced with compassion, love and prayer. We must keep in mind that there are always two sides to the truth in human matters. The universal truth is, that which we consider bad is God, and that which we consider good is God: this is the whole of God as He manifests in the world.

The first refinement of higher consciousness is to accept the presence of God in darkness as well as in light. All situations are opportunities for growth that prepare us for the future. With a telescopic, neutral mind we are able to see the opportunities hidden in the challenges we encounter. By finding our faith in each of life's moments we find love. A True Spiritual Master will teach that God enters on the wings of Love, Faith and Hope, and helps us see through to the heart of any matter. Only with Divine Love are we able to heal ourselves and effectively communicate with others to reach their hearts. As we walk through life imperfectly, we are given the chance to evolve. The healthiest change is brought about in evolution, and not in revolution. A true living Master will teach that we are all incarnations of God who must be approached with tolerance and grace.

A Naam Yogi must lead by example. As you face your obstacles and complications with tolerance, compassion and spiritual transcendence, you give others permission to do the same. As you acknowledge how to utilize the ego in the service of fortifying right action and aligning with the Divine, you will become an earthly representative of Heaven. If you desire to open your heart and see the unseen, then find a Master who sees the unseen so that he may give you the correct method of working with Naam in order to help you lift the veil. Read this book, along with *Lifting the Veil, Alchemy of Love Relationships, The Divine Doctor* and *The Healing Fire of Heaven* for Wisdom, Life, Love, Health and Light; vibrate Naam; and recite the *Prayer of Love, Peace and Light* (see page 216). The luminous beings in the entire cosmos are all indebted to us because of the *Prayer of Love, Peace and Light*. Let's make this prayer the foundation of all our lives. There is greatness in store for those who practice Naam Yoga and recite this prayer on a daily basis with sincerity and the intention to spread these qualities throughout the universe. Again, finding and working with a True Spiritual Master who sees the unseen is the highest blessing that you can receive from God while living on earth.

INTRODUCTION

THE PRACTICE OF NAAM is the highest, most beautiful and most powerful spiritual practice. The simplicity of this heavenly path is not in ritualism. Rather, it is in the reality of practicing with the Word so that the one who has no love can have love; the one who has no faith can have faith; the one who has no hope can have hope.

The Word is the greatest power on the planet. There was, is, and never shall be anything beyond it. No other power can compare to that of the Word, for the Word is the basis, the giver, of all life. It is the first cause, the projected God. By the power of the Word, in the Word, and through the Word, all things, both seen and unseen, have been created.

The Word is the creative power of the primal light and the universal key that unlocks the fifty gates of life. The Kabbalah Tree of Life has ten Sephiroth. Each Sephirah also has five divisions. Ten times five equals fifty. Thus, the Kabbalah speaks of fifty gates of intelligence or understanding. These fifty gates of intelligence and understanding are symbolically attributed to Binah. In order to open the Sephirah and make yourself privy to the knowledge and understanding that lies therein, you need a key. The key is self-knowledge and self-healing. One needs the master key of self knowledge that the Word bestows to open these gates. With this key, you can know everything, for when you know yourself, you know the entire universe. You can open the gates of all the regions of heaven. As both the beginning of all and the power by which everything is created, the Word represents all that is creative, positive, and healing. Working with the Word, then, is the most secret and powerful practice known to yogis and Kabbalists. The truth of the matter is that practicing the 84 yoga postures will lengthen your physical life, but they will not open your heart and bind you with God. God is bound by the Word, whose existence serves to keep the universe in balance. It is through the practice of the Word—the true essence of divinity, root of all things, and nucleus of spiritual energy, that man is able to merge with God. This is the highest practice of any form of spirituality and healing, including Kabbalah and yoga. Through the use of the Word students of Universal Kabbalah become new people. The Word recharges their systems and empowers their minds, thereby accelerating their potential for excellence. As the antidote to depression and repairer of the nervous system, the Word grounds you in who you really are by developing your relationship with your pranic body. It bestows the capacity to deal with life resolutely. Understand that nothing is equal to the power of the Word. Only the mantric way can truly elevate the self beyond duality and establish the flow of the spirit. Practicing with the Word will enable you to acknowledge the splendor of God present in all things, while simultaneously permitting the Divine to speak to you through your reality in order to guide and reassure you.

The Universal Kabbalist is able to realize his/her oneness with the universe and gain access to universal knowledge via the use of mantric prayer and through the power of the Word. Through consistent practice and application of the Word, he/she begins to realize that the power that has held him/her in bondage is the very power that, when properly directed, can free him/her. How does the Word accomplish this? The power of the Word is a projected combination tuned to create certain vibratory effects in the mind and body. Indeed, mantric prayer is the science of shifting from one frequency to another. Therefore, the use of the Word is the ultimate method available for tuning the mind. It is the essence, the projection, the destiny, and the art of bringing new life to the individual. Understand that all power derives from the Word, and not human beings. The sound of the vibration of the Word is all that you are to master, for vibration holds all of the Universe and every dimension. He who knows the law of vibrations knows the whole secret of life. The power of the Word is all-dimensional and, as such, is internal as well as external. It bestows the power to tap into the unknown. When all energy and matter is synchronized into a point, it is infinity, and infinity does not know defeat. The ecstasy of the power of the Word that was in the beginning, which is now, and which shall ever be, is always with us.

All beginnings, all seeds, all things come from the Word. This sacred practice will put hope in your soul, faith in your spirit, and love in your heart, and you will see the beauty and light of life, and the entire heavens will speak to you. By vibrating the Word, one releases wondrous forces within himself and in his surroundings. When these forces mix with the application of the Divine Spiritual Wisdom, they create the alchemy that works miracles. The benefits of such a practice are many. The mind becomes so pure and radiantly healthy it can even cause a sick body to regain balance and vitality. This is the secret of the sages. To fight or escape disease they use the spiritual device of the Word, for they know that the Word is the panacea that cures all ills. The practice of the Word increases the thickness in cortical regions of the brain related to sensory, auditory and visual perception, as well as internal perception and the automatic monitoring of heart rate, or breathing.

Regular practice of chanting prayer also slows age-related thinning of the frontal cortex. Pain causes an unexpected brain drain; pain and stress cause the brain to shrink. People in constant pain lose gray matter equal to an oversized pea each year. Gray matter is an outer layer of the brain rich in nerve cells and crucial to information and memory processing. Stress and pain cause a degradation of our neurons, which are the signal transmitters of the mind and body. The neurons become overactive or overstressed from activity. People born with smaller numbers of neurons are predisposed to suffering from chronic pain. There is a direct correlation between brain volume and intelligence. IQ is not only related to the amount of gray matter in the brain, but it is also distributed throughout the brain, rather than being localized in one area. In general, men think more with their gray matter and women tend to rely more on white matter, the other primary type of brain tissue. The Word is a cosmic contained energy which revitalizes those who work with it. Vibrating it is the best way to become free of disease.

Working with the Divine Spiritual Wisdom in conjunction with the Word also bestows spiritual growth. As you move into a state of physical and mental health and blossom spiritually, you are then able to help heal others through the power of the Word. Indeed, the very touch of one who has mastered the practice of the Word can drive disease away. The one who works with the Divine Spiritual Wisdom and has merged with the Word is like the philosopher's stone, and those who are within the orbit and aura of his potent influence become healthy and happy. Indeed, the only sure path to happiness is the Word, for it opens the heart and grants wisdom, light, kindness, and grace. On the Kabbalah Tree of Life, you will find the creative Word under the Sephirah Chokmah. And the name of God in the sphere Chokmah is *Yah*. His servant is *Raziel*, the mystery of God, the Archangel of life, knowledge, wisdom, and the power of the Divine Word. Raziel commands the Ophanim, known as Cherubim in the Christian tradition, who watch over the harmony of the cosmos under the authority of the Word. Their empire is immense, stretching all the way to the zodiac, known in Hebrew as Mazaloth. In other words, its astrological attribution refers to the wheel of the zodiac, revealing its supraterrestrial sphere of influence.

Those who work with the Word, then, possess the key that opens all doors and enables the practitioner to accomplish the miraculous, first within himself, then within others, and finally within the whole of nature. It will cause you to utilize the physical structure of your present form in perfect harmony with the energetic structure of your soul to bring about the great potential for the expression and expansion of light through your being. Man's creativity is potentially infinite. The entire self-creativity can be expanded and experienced by working with the Word. God created man simply to reveal himself in the finite as infinity. The Word will bring you in harmony with your origin and your originality. The Word is a golden key that causes you to find your soul, and you realize that your soul is nothing but a projection of God Almighty, which is love, and that love is everywhere in your consciousness. As a result, you speak through the tongue, the identity of the light, so that darkness may be removed and light may be spread. For a human, in his essence, is with infinite, unlimited creative power some people call God.

If man goes within himself and consciously experiences his own beauty, he becomes God. Practice of the Word gives you beauty, bounty, bliss, and virtue. The Word causes you to find Purkha in you, so that you may live by Prakirti. When nature and you become one, you become divine. You become One. Those who practice with the Word are the last key of the time psycho-electromagnetic field of the psyche of the individual birth planet. They will cover the fifth calendar of the zodiac. While other eras have been two thousand years, they have been given three thousand in which to elaborate their existence.

The electromagnetic field of the planet supports the fact that those who practice with the Word shall come to rule the planet. The Word of the living God is beginning to be heard, and it will transform everything. Therefore, for us to feel comfortable, the immortal principal within must expand and absorb the corruptible principle without so that the envelope of the senses may be lifted, and we can appear in our pristine purity. This process is achieved through a true opening of the heart, via the Word, and the development of the internal organ that allows us to receive God. Upon completion of the process whereby we open our hearts and develop our internal spiritual organ, the metaphysical and incorruptible principle comes to rule over the terrestrial principle and human beings, filled with the light of heaven, begin to experience the grace and joy from above. By the power of the Word, all known and unknown negativity, including death, leaves. Learn this sacred science and it will protect you by healing all sorrows, removing all suffering, and destroying all disease, for the power of the Word is no small thing. It is a revitalizing, manifested power, cosmic energy contained, and the direct dialing code between the finite and the Infinite. By working with the Word we can regain our pristine power which we lost since the Fall of Man.

Before the Fall, human beings had the faculty to perceive and understand the hidden, eternal truths via an inner spiritual organ. This organ was given to us as a result of our incorruptibility and immortality. After the Fall, when we rendered ourselves mortal and corruptible, we received the outer organs we now call the five senses. This envelope of senses is truly a corruptible substance found in our blood, forming the fleshly bonds that bind our immortal spirits, making them the servants of our mortal flesh. Indeed, at present, our inner faculty is enveloped in gross matter to the extent that the external eye cannot see into the spiritual realms, we are deaf to the sounds of the metaphysical world, and our speech has been paralyzed so that we can barely stammer the words of sacred import. These are the words that were once ours, and through them we held sway over the elemental forces and the external world. Therefore, we must learn the heavenly science and work with the Word, in order to develop the lost inner faculty that allows us to perceive the hidden, eternal truths. Otherwise one will not find fulfillment. No external comfort in this world can give us the fulfillment we crave. No amount of riches and power can ultimately satiate our hearts; man has been a creature enslaved by his own mind and ego to sow dissatisfaction throughout his life and throughout the lives of others. We use the human form, which was granted to us for the sublime purpose of God realization, to tyrannize other living beings through misuse of will, rendering our state worse than that of the best.

When we operate from the ego, we are not our true selves; we are controlling our lives via our mind. The mind does not like simple things; it loves to complicate everything and render the simplest of tasks difficult. The mind distracts us to follow many paths, so that no destination may be reached. It also makes us quick to complain, whereas the heart naturally makes us grateful. When we are mired in our minds, we find fault with everyone: those who are blessed with work complain about their jobs. Married couples complain of distress within the relationship; unmarried people complain they have not found the right partner. Others complain of unemployment and poverty, disease and death. The mind will even complain simultaneously of that which it possesses and that which it does not possess. Universal law shows us that when we do not feel gratitude for something, it will be taken away, so that through the pain of separation, the individual realizes that he has been separating himself from God. For the sustainer of the self is God. Remembering to feel gratitude connects us directly with the divine. Furthermore, when we give freely without conditions, we become the action of God and feel even more connected and more blessed.

Everywhere we turn, a tide of pain, misery, and grief seems to be engulfing mankind. However, if we examine the cause of this worldwide discord, we discover that we are actually the architects of our own suffering. When we constantly feed negative thoughts into the engine of the mind, we cause immense harm not only to ourselves, but we also affect world consciousness. A slip of the mind in terms of negative thinking is, in fact, a slip of our destiny. And if we rely only on our minds, which are allied with the ego, we have no chance except to wrestle with our internal wild horses that wish to break free. The suffering of the world is neither in the soul nor in the body; it is in our mind. The soul is the friend of the body; our soul is the pure essence of life, and our body is the circumference of life. Your mind exists between your body and your soul. It is your friend and servant, not your master. He who considers the mind his master shall never find his true master. Life is given to you to experience through the process of mind which is the perceiver, the joy of life. Yet, we must train the wild horses of the mind by opening our hearts, honoring our life will, freeing ourselves of the tyranny of the mind. The mind then will become secondary to the heart, and life will be nothing but beauty and happiness.

We are living in a foreign land. As this world is not our True Home, our time here is merely a transitory phase of life. While this world, and all it contains, is impermanent, we associate with it as if we belong to it, and it belongs to us. Understand that matter and mind are constructed from the five elements, or tattvas: earth, water, fire, air, and akasha. (Akasha is the matter that surrounds the earth beyond air, and is often called ether.) These five tattvas join to become something and disintegrate to become nothing. This explains the conventional concept of life and death, and it is in this way that one can evaporate and reform.

Our journey on this earth is an experience of polarity that no one is above. The earth has a north and a south pole, and you see both your self and your shadow. Just as the soul of Archetypal Man is a prisoner of Universal Matter, so too is the soul of each individual a prisoner of his physical body. In reality the individual soul is an essence of the Ocean of Light and Bliss, pure, radiant, and transcendent. It is a drop of the ocean of eternal happiness. But, through its age-old association with the mind, the soul has gathered so much base impurity that it has completely forgotten its origin. It has become burdened by the mind, an organ led by the five senses, and has come to believe that this world is its real abode. The soul suffers the material consequences of this unfortunate association, and has to go through the long cycle of life and death. Upon death, the elements are absorbed back into the Tattvas, the mind is absorbed into the Universal Mind, and the soul is absorbed into the Infinite Soul. The reincarnations that follow physical death are the means through which the fallen entities exercise their control over man. Reintegration is the only way to escape the cycles of reincarnation.

The Wisdom, Strength, and Beauty that are still manifesting in this material universe are the efforts of Archetypal Man to regain the position he occupied before the Fall. Meanwhile, opposite qualities are being manifested by the fallen entities. This is their attempt to maintain the climate that they created, so that they could exist as they wanted when they refused to re-enter Omneity. Man will not regain his first splendor and freedom unless he separates himself from the lower three chakras, for it is via these chakras that the fallen entities exercise their control and bind him. The fallen entities, however, are constantly fighting man's tendency towards perfection by tempting him so as to keep him confined to this world.

Unfortunately, because man has to descend into the material world, where he is constantly breathing the fruits of his malefic intellect, he is in a bad position to resist the constant temptations of the three lower chakras. Fortunately, the Creator re-established the equilibrium by detaching from His Spiritual Divine Circle a Major Spirit to act as guide, counselor, and companion of the Minor who descends from the celestial immensity to be incorporated into the material world and to work, according to his free will, on the earth plane.

While the fact that we are in human form signifies that we have fallen, it is only in human form that the soul can come into contact with a master in order to get the secret of the lost Word. Once the secret of the lost Word has been retrieved and devotedly practiced, the soul attains liberation. Practicing the eighty-four postures of yoga will lengthen your life, but the practice of the Word is vital to Fallen Man, for it bestows the mysterious ordination that is the vital condition of man's reconciliation. Without the Word, man will remain in privation without true communication with God, no matter how great his personal merits.

The ability to receive and work with the Word is a privilege reserved for man alone. No other species has this ability. Amongst all the beings that inhabit the Earth, we are the only ones who are endowed with the full power of speech and, therefore, the Word. In other words, it is only in the human form that the soul can realize God and retrace its footsteps back to its original Home. The human body, then, becomes the vehicle whereby one can be released from the vast prison of pain and misery, of evolution and de-evolution. The problem is that, as human beings, our minds have become so feeble and erring that we are unable to resist sensory pleasures. Easily falling prey to such temptations, we ultimately become trapped in an unending cycle of want and desire. Even as our minds realize that the outcome of all over-indulgence in sense enjoyment is pain, sorrow, and dejection, it persists in its pursuit.

To escape the cycles of reincarnation in this infernal world, man must detach himself from everything that attracts him to matter, and disengage from the slavery of the three lower centers and material sensations. He also has to elevate himself morally. In order to do so, man must constantly fight against the fallen entities by unmasking and rejecting them from his domain. This is achieved in two ways. Firstly, through initiation, which attaches him to the elements of the already reunited Archetypes that constitute the exoteric communion of Saints. Secondly, through the liberating knowledge that comes from the Divine Spiritual Wisdom that teaches him the means of self-healing and enhancement of his personal work as well as the means of helping, uplifting, and serving the rest of humanity.

It is only after individual liberation that the great collective liberation will take place. The great collective liberation will allow the reconstitution of the Archetype and its reintegration into the Divine. Abandoned by its animator and left under the anarchic nature of the fallen spirits, the material world will dissolve at an accelerated pace. The end of the physical universe, as announced by the great traditions, will then take place.

If we understand that every action has an equal reaction, and that the wise among us keep the end result of any action in their sights, why do we persist in adopting the insane course of constantly striving to fulfill our sensory pleasures? Better still, how do we keep our minds from continually re-engaging in such a circular trap? In order to find a suitable remedy we must consider the nature of the mind. It is fond of pleasure, and can never seem to settle in stillness on one thing. Rather, it flits from one idea, notion, and thing to another as soon as it detects something it deems sweeter than what it already has. In so doing, it destroys what it has in hand. Like love and attraction, the mind is never constant.

There is a spiritual science which allows you to make the brain work in such a way as to clear our subconscious mind of negativity, so that we may live from our heart. How much it takes for a person to rise above the clouds depends on how much he can consciously guide the subconscious mind. For a human being is sixty-percent water, the mind is like the moon and our thoughts are like waves on an ocean. As the moon creates tides in the ocean, so does the mind create tides of vibration in the human body. When our thoughts are channeled and stilled, there are no tides. Then, the mind becomes cool and calm, in a state of deep meditation. If we consider that physical health is the sustainer of life, then our mental health may be considered as the essence of life. Therefore, the mind is the horse that you have to ride in order to reach your destiny. The mind is an energy, it is not the self. It is a horse that you need to break, so that it may gracefully take you through time and space. Due to the mind's fickleness, it will readily give up all if we provide it with something sweeter and more absorbing than worldly pleasures. That something is within us, within our bodies. It is resounding above and behind our eyes in the form of the sweet music the saints call *Shabad*, mantra, the Word, Sound Current or Audible Life Stream. The science of the Word has been lost to most of humankind. When we fell from the Garden of Eden, Man lost his capacity of knowing and hearing the Word from heaven that cure all illnesses and bring eternal life, as represented by the Tree of Life. We became receptive to the words that were uttered below the earth, and sacrificed the Word from heaven. Many holy scriptures give evidence of the power of the Word; human beings have often chosen to believe the spirit of the Word rather than honor a deeper truth contained therein.

The Divine Spiritual Wisdom is hidden in all the scriptures of the world. It must be practiced and experienced so that the knowledge is not lost for the coming generations. By the practice of the Word through mantra, the mind gives in, and man merges with God. Mantra is the vibration that ushers in the power of the Sun, as well as the limitless power of creativity. When the mind truly hears this celestial music, all worldly pleasures become tasteless. Indeed, there is no power on this planet greater than the Word. The Word serves to keep the universe in balance. Without it, the universe would fall apart and disappear. It is by the power of Word, in the Word, and through the Word that all things, both seen and unseen, have been created. There was, is, and never shall be anything beyond it. God is bound by the Word and, therefore, the Word has the power to bring us to God.

The sounds we utter are produced when our tongue touches various points in the mouth at the same time that the lips are opening and closing. Sounds then group together to make words with different meanings, conveyed in both the words themselves and their modes of expression. This process gradually transforms the music of sound into language. Music can exist independently of language, but language can never free itself from music.

A key difference between creating a word and creating a sound lies in the application of the breath. A word is a more pronounced utterance of breath fashioned by the mouth and tongue. It is in the capacity of the mouth that breath then becomes voice. Therefore, the original condition of a word is breath. In this way, the saying "First was the breath" is synonymous with the saying "In the beginning was the Word." The voice is an interesting indication of an individual's characteristics. The depth of one's tone reveals the level of strength and power, while the height of one's pitch expresses love and wisdom. We convey a variety of sentiments—sincerity, insincerity, inclination, disinclination, pleasure, and displeasure with the variety of our musical expressions.

With a thorough knowledge of which mantras alleviate certain conditions, a Master gives mantras—an elite combination of both language and music—to his students in the same way a physician prescribes medication. Students are often asked to repeat certain mantras for a specific amount of time and days. This is due to the fact that numbers are a science, and each number of repetitions has a unique value. Indeed, it is in repetition that the secret of power lays. Mystics, therefore, give great importance to the number of repetitions. Just as a lower dose of a certain medicine may heal, while a higher dose of the same medicine may kill, a single mantric repetition means one thing, while a few repetitions means something quite different.

Understand that when Christ commanded that we abstain from vain repetitions he was not, as is often thought, referring to the sacred name as used in worship or religious practices.

We live, and move, and have our very being in God. All forms of worship and/or belief should draw one closer to God. That which separates man from God has no value. When man is separated from God in thought, neither his beliefs nor his worship is of any use.

Remember the refrain, "In the beginning was the Word, and the Word was with God, and the Word was God." As we work with the Word via chanting prayer, God becomes our rock and our protective shield. In Him we take refuge. Those who master the Word receive the Lord's shield of salvation and His sustaining right hand. His gentleness makes them great. To be sure, the Most High will arm us with strength and make our way perfect, subduing those who seek to rise up against us and rescuing us from our enemies. *Triple Mantra* is particularly effective in this regard, as it allows God to create a shield of defense around us. With consistent practice, we can walk through the valley of the shadow of death, fearing no evil, for we know that the Light of God is with us. Use the Word and the Lord shall be your shepherd. The King of Glory will come into every aspect of your life, restoring your soul so that you lack nothing. Your cup shall runneth over, and goodness and kindness shall follow you all the days of your life as His name guides you on the path of righteousness. Use the Word, and let the Heaven pluck you from the net that has been laid secretly by negative forces.

Those who master the Word shall inherit the land, and shall delight in the abundance of peace. God is the King of the Earth, and blessed is the person who practices the Word and makes HIM his trust. Through mantra, we must ask Heaven to purify us so that we may be clean; to wash us so that we may be whiter than snow; to grant us a pure heart; to renew us with right spirit; to restore us with the joy of His salvation. Chanting prayer allows one to emanate life in such a way that it reveals everything to you, and opens all the doors to you. It opens your inner eyes and ears, and you begin to see the invisible realities.

All knowledge of the divine, spiritual, and physical worlds will come to those who work with the Divine Spiritual Wisdom via the Word. By working with the Word, you are saying, "Lord, I want to do your will, not mine. Come and dwell within me, I have prepared a place for you." When you trust in the Word, and the Lord's way for you, everything in your life begins to fall into place. You begin to dwell in the shelter of the Most High and to rest in the shadow of the Almighty. But, you must be willing to turn yourself over completely, and give God a chance. If, through the use of the sound current, you make the Most High your dwelling place, no harm will befall you. Indeed, the day you realize that the Word is God and God is the Word, and decide to place God at the head of your life, the Archangels of the Lord will guard you, and the Angels will lift you up in their hands so that you may gracefully move through the challenges of time and space. Therefore, practice with the Word and let God be your high tower.

Working with mantra is the inner way. It is an inside job. It is the way of prayer and the way of the heart, and the fastest way to unite with the Divine. The yoga of Pranayam (breathing) cannot take us beyond the six centers. Only Naad Yoga, the Yoga of the Audible Life Stream, mantra yoga, the Word or Logos of the Bible, can take us to the Highest Region, which is Eternal. Again, the more you unite with the divine Source, the more help and support you will attract. Through the assistance you receive, you become strong and radiant. You take control of yourself, and come to possess the powerful keys to realization. The only thing you have to fear is that you will commit an act that sends the Luminous Beings from your midst. Remember, each fault produces dark, sickening emanations that these Luminous Beings cannot stand. The thing that attracts them is the pure, harmonious ambiance created by the one who chants consistently in the early morning hours and, therefore, places God at the center of his or her life. All riches and powers do not give us fulfillment and satisfaction. It is the awakening of the soul and the true opening of the heart which does.

The head creates the illusion that wisdom resides within it, when in fact, wisdom comes from the heart. Human beings have been given intellect with which to reason, but wisdom has been bestowed upon us by the Divine, and therefore is locked within the heart. The key to understanding this wisdom lies in the mystery of the Word. When an individual learns about divine spiritual matters under the direction of a master who comprehends this golden path, a great power is released within his heart, which begins to open and to heal itself, eliminating ill will to others and strengthening his entire being.

The divine science uses the repetition of the proper sacred words to appeal to the heavens and bring about the desired result. Each vowel has a psychological meaning, and the composition of every word has a chemical and psychological significance that is connected to astrological science and the Kabbalah. For example, we may use a certain word to evoke a planet in the cosmos, either to diminish its influence on our endeavors if it is blocking our path or to increase its power in our lives if it is favorable to us. Yogis and Kabbalists repeat certain words to achieve illumination. This is a sublime science. Chanting prayer stimulates the upper palate with the tip of the tongue, tuning the thalamus and hypothalamus. Focusing on the tip of the nose causes our frontal lobe, which controls our personality, to become like lead. At one point the pain can become so unbearable, making it a bit difficult to stand it until it breaks. As a result, you have found what you are looking for, and it is yours forever. No one can take it away from you.

The destiny of every human being is written on his forehead; behind it resides the brain, which contains the divine glands, commonly called the pituitary and pineal glands. The third eye, called the Agna chakra, also resides within the confines of the forehead, and is considered the command headquarters of the entire consciousness of all human beings. When we chant, we stimulate the divine glands to heal all areas of the body, as well as clear out karma and create a new path for our spiritual future. Prayer is the ultimate power, and that power is in you.

Our sacred science leads to Christic consciousness. It shows the way to illumination. It gives you the blessings of happiness and health while on earth. It gives you that pure energy which activates the inner faculty of the spiritual and incorruptible body, putting you in direct contact with the higher world, and all things start to work automatically. Nothing will properly work in your life until you activate this interior faculty of your immortal body. It moves the energy from your Silver cord to your Gold cord and you get Superconsciousness in Consciousness.

It is important that you do not spend much time worrying yourself over how to sort things out on the physical plane. The physical plane is the world of consequences, and over which we have very little power. Instead of addressing the world of consequences, we must strive to address the world of causes. This is the only way to bring about lasting change, for it is there that we have all the means to contact and trigger the beneficial forces that will, sooner or later, produce some positive results in our lives. But, most people do not know this. Their minds tell them that they must intervene on the physical plane. These people are continually surprised that the material changes they seek to bring about do not last. Events or people come to shake things up, and in the end, they remain no more in control of a given situation than they were before. Do not partake in this scenario in your own life. If, for example, you want to change your habits, tackle them by chanting. This is the best way to rise through thought to the causal plane to be united with wisdom, love, and truth. With the release of such power comes change on the physical plane. No change is possible or worthwhile unless it changes the spiritual foundation. That is the base. One must work at the base and build it up. Attacking the physical plane to create a change is called patchwork. Patchwork will never bring you lasting satisfaction. The mantric way, or Naad yoga, is the science of syllables which open your base, your naadis (energy channels in the body), changing your chemistry. For mantra is the power of manifestation, which takes the human mind and heart to an experience of its origin in the creator and bestows the experience of divine ecstasy—the ecstasy that brings harmony in every aspect of life.

Sound is not only the mother of Light, it also creates life, moving one from darkness to light, from duality to divinity. It is the healing love that flows from heaven. By mastering a mantram, or the holy Naam, we move from the gross to the subtle, and from the subtle to the infinite. Understand that mantra yoga, the science of union with the higher consciousness, is not a new science. It has existed since the beginning of time. Indeed, all saints and sages testify that God is within our hearts, and that our sorrows and worries will cease only when we turn our attention inward. Indeed, those we revere as saints did not come to establish a new religion, nor a new creed, nor even a new sect. Their mission is simply to liberate the qualified souls, through the power of the Word, from this land of misery, guiding them back to their Home of Eternal Bliss and Peace.

The God-realization of which we speak is not possible without a Master who sees the unseen. Only a Master can show you how to vacate the nine portals of the body in order to fully enter the tenth portal leading to the Eternal Home. This is not so unusual when we consider that each of us needs a teacher at every stage of life. Your first guru is your mother. She teaches you how to sit, stand, walk, eat, drink, and dress. Later, your father, mother, brothers, and sisters teach you how to speak. As you grow older, your friends and playmates teach you the art of social interaction. At school, your teachers teach you the skills of learning. You can determine, then, how necessary it is that a guru teaches you the science of the soul.

Not only is it impossible to know God without the help of a true initiate, it is also potentially dangerous. Without a guide, we are sure to lose our way and fall into a quagmire of delusion and danger. The Perfect Master will show us how and where to enter the body, the temple of the living God. As previously stated, there are nine outlets that lead to the sense world, but only the tenth outlet opens into the spiritual regions. This is called the Sushumna gate, which is located in the center of the forehead, behind the eyes. It is through this aperture that we pass beyond matter and mind to reach the Everlasting and Immortal.

This path, the path of the saints, does not ask you to give up on life in the material world. You are not required to renounce religion, family, friends, or your mode of living. Indeed, you are to live in the world, but sensibly. Enjoy it, walk in the material garden, enjoying its fruits, but realize its true worth. The objects, situations, and circumstances of this world are here to serve you. Use them, but do not allow yourself to be used by them. In other words, guard against permitting your mind to become so entangled in attachments that they enslave you. Be in the world, but not of it. The only requirement is that you devote some time, daily and punctually to the most important of your earthly duties, namely, practice of devotion to God and listening to His voice, that Celestial Sound within. For, you can do all the meditating, worshipping and performing rituals, but it will not be real until you find the Word. The Word is your own identity. The Word will give you your own truth. Your own truth will give you endurance, tolerance, grace and competency. Without it, you will build your expectations on someone or something else, and these expectations never come true. Your true work in this life is that of keeping up with your spiritual discipline. If you keep up, and trust in the process, it will, in due course, liberate you from the vast prison in which you have been confined for countless ages. Time is fleeting, and physical life is short. Take full advantage of the life you have while it is still yours. If you have not done your own work already, start doing it now. Seek a true Master and under his guidance attach your soul to the Word, and reach your True Home.

As you learn the Divine Spiritual Wisdom and practice the sacred words (mantra) revealed on the Rootlight CD series, you will generate a healing energy that will extend for a 25-mile radius (even farther for those who possess high levels of consciousness, such as masters). This explains why the work of highly evolved beings alone can benefit an entire city or sometimes a country. If you practice mantra, you will wipe out all karmas previously created, neutralizing your being and casting out negativity and depression. When mantra is practiced in a group or during class under the direction of one who practices and reveres the power of the Word, the psychic and inner unfoldment of everyone in that group is greatly increased, because an atmosphere of higher etheric vibrations is created in an environment. Indeed, a beneficial atmosphere of higher etheric vibrations is created in an environment where mantra is being chanted, because when 100 people chant mantra, and 100 people hear it, you square the whole thing and you get the power of 10,000. The concentrated and highly charged vibrations of such a harmonious group attracts to it heavenly vibrations of great potency, resulting in an increased stimulation of all our spiritual faculties.

To clarify, a mantra is a series of sounds that have been designed to elevate or modify the consciousness through rhythmic repetition. Its power is not so much in the meaning of the words, but rather in the pattern of the vibrations it creates. Under vibration, small particles of matter group together in a definite geometric pattern and/or figure that corresponds to the quality, strength, and rhythm of the sound. At the vibratory level, sound creates light. Because each color has a life sound, and each sound a form color, all mantras have a corresponding color and form. In other words, matter and energy are dependent on light, and light is dependent on sound. Each of the coded sounds found within mantra has a unique vibratory effect that can help you find and keep your center. Each mantra implants a positive affirmation in your psyche. This is the divine thought-medicine for the mind that allows for healing what experience and karma has shattered. By chanting mantra, we are performing *Japa*, the act of calling on energy that is beyond us. We are connecting to the Lord through the power of our thought waves.

As you employ your tongue to chant mantra, your consciousness is positively affected. The tongue is a precious tool that comes from the central vagus nerve. It is responsible for many events in our lives, both happy and unhappy. Through the use, or misuse, of our tongues, we win or lose friends. It takes a long time to build something and it takes one moment to destroy anything. A slip of the tongue can destroy your whole life. You must realize that the tongue was not given to man to be used to weaken or destroy others. It was given to man to heal and uplift others. It's primary function is to help the one who has fallen, to enlighten and encourage the one who is searching for the Divine Spiritual Wisdom, to guide the one who is lost, and to uplift humankind. Therefore, employ your tongue wisely. Use it to bless, heal, give thanks, and enliven others.

God sits at the tip of your tongue. Use it to bring the harmony of the heavens around you. Those who do not understand the value of right speech and the folly of slander will eventually, in this life or the next, lose the ability of their tongues. For those wicked who have sharpened their tongues like a serpent, and the viper's poison is under their lips, will be thrown into the karmic fire, the miry pits from whence they shall never rise. Understand that those whose tongues plot deceitful destruction, rather than peace, love evil more than they love good. They lie rather than speak the truth, and their lies devour. They judge blamelessly and, in their hearts, plot injustice. They are poison, and their own tongues shall be their ruin. At the right time, the Lord of karma will destroy them forever. He will pluck them from their tents, rooting them out of the land of the living. As the righteous ones see this, they will come to understand how divine justice works to wash the wicked away. Those who do not connect with God in order to trust in the abundance of their riches and strengthen themselves against their own wickedness, shall soon regret it.

This universe is an electromagnetic field. It has a longitude and latitude of magnetic wavelengths. Therefore, this comic universe is very communicative, it talks to us. In this talk, all personalities are built and marred. Therefore, one should always speak very carefully, consciously, and intelligently knowing what that shall mean to Infinity. Remember the Word is God and God is the Word. You are what your words are. The time has come for people to understand the sacredness of the tongue. Pray with your tongue. As you employ your tongue to chant mantra, your consciousness is positively affected. In essence, you are going into intercourse with the higher worlds. Chanting raises you inwardly to the higher planes. The mouth functions as the uterus, and the tongue functions as the male organ. The mouth, then, is the *Gian guphaa*, or wisdom cave. This royal yoga causes the pituitary and pineal glands to secrete faster than any other practice. And, the purpose of all spiritual practice is to create that secretion. There are eighty-four meridian points that one can stimulate with the tongue on the upper palate of the human mouth. There are two rows of meridian points, eighty-four on the upper palate. Through the practice of chanting prayer the tongue stimulates these meridian points, which is the base of the brain. They in turn stimulate the hypothalamus, which makes the pineal glands radiate. When the pineal gland radiates, it creates an impulsation in the pituitary gland. When the pituitary gives the impulsation, the entire glandular system secretes and a human being obtains bliss. Then consciousness can be achieved. This is the science. Chant mantra, and God will shield you from the conspiracy of the wicked ones and the noisy clamor of evildoers.

Chanting prayer exalts the mind, inspiring an indissoluble unity with God. That is what chanting prayer achieves. The pathway of prayer is the practice of the Word, which creates the vibratory sound current that opens up the *Trikutee*, the inner center of the brain that, when stimulated, gives us the experience of ecstasy. *Naam*, which means God's name, or the Word, leads us to *Naad*, the sound current. Naad takes us to *Aad*, which means the beginning—God, or Infinity. The Word is the key to the mystery of the whole life, the mystery of all planes of existence. There is nothing that cannot be accomplished, there is nothing that cannot be known, by the power of the word. The key to the true path of light is the Word.

The deeper we dive into the mystery of life, the more we discover that its entire secret is hidden in words. All spiritual science and practices are based upon the science of sound. All language has a mantric quality. The words we use everyday are, in effect, low-grade mantras that connect us to the lower world and the beast within. Know that between what you communicate and what is communicated to you, the pattern of your lifestyle is created and computed in your subconscious mind. In turn, you become whatever your subconscious mind process is. There are words which are powerful based on their meaning, others because of the vibration they produce, and others due to their influence on various centers of the brain. These words have been given to saints, sages, and prophets through inspirations from God; within them is concealed precious information of how to acquire all that the soul yearns for in life. When we meditate daily, dwelling upon a mantra or prayer given to us by a spiritually enlightened person, one who knows God in intimate communion, we attain a sympathetic understanding and devotion, and our minds will be exalted to similar heights of spiritual discernment. The phenomenon of sympathetic vibration will awaken us to a realization of the Divine consciousness within us, in a holy and mystical experience. The mantras we chant in accordance with the divine sacred wisdom connect us to the higher worlds and our higher selves. Chanting prayer brings in us the absolute redemption from karma. In truth, the destiny of a person is written in the Word, by repeating the Divine Word, one can change their fate and fulfill their highest destiny. The practice of the Word through mantra will renew your cells and awaken faculties within you whose existence you have never been aware of. A daily communion with the Word will make your life luminous, spiritual and pure.

The mantric way is the method of training the divine one, and the method by which the new spiritual body we will inhabit will be organized. We pray so that the Christic principle that lies dormant within us may be awakened and illuminate our consciousness, for the light of God is the living principle of human life. We are the radiance; the light of God, and our future lies in the light of infinity, which is God.

When, without hesitation or doubt, you direct your mind and heart toward the divine, you are demonstrating your love of God in prayer. Your prayer, your call to the sky, establishes a bond with the cosmic via the luminous beings that invisibly assist us in realizing our legitimate desires. The magical and intimate experience of bonding with the cosmic reveals all hidden things so that you come to understand the meaning of life. Prayer, then, is the spiritual technology that aligns us with the divine and allows us to solve the most difficult of dilemmas. Indeed, when we truly endeavor to love God, to adore Him, to honor Him with contrition of heart, to invoke him in all matters which we wish to undertake, and to operate with very great devotion, God will lead us in the right way and reward us with success.

Mantras, or sound currents, along with spiritual symbols, hold the inner and holy truth. The mantric way leads to the process of regeneration, or spiritual birth. The regenerated soul, which results from a union of the conscious, the emotional, and the intellectual, is a purely spiritual offspring of the union of the spirit and body. True regeneration, then, acts on both the spiritual and physical vehicles to awaken and renew the soul powers. Right speaking, thinking, and acting renews the cells and tissues of the physical body, raising them to a higher state of vibration so that they are better able to coordinate their functions with the spiritual vehicle. When we consider that regeneration is the process of renewing, recreating, and reproducing latent soul powers from a part of the complete individual by the action of the spiritual vehicle of man, we come to understand that regeneration actually reproduces and renews a new organism from a portion of the complete individual.

As we said earlier, the practice of mantra, the practice of true prayer, prepares us properly for the worship of God in spirit and in truth. It is the science of rebinding man with God that brings about the accomplishment of beneficial changes in our fundamental state of being. These changes then allow us to become the servants of the universe or agents of God who bring those who are guided by their heads and led by the turbulence of passion to the ways of Peace, Light, and Wisdom.

Everything lies in the mind. It is your control center. With eyes nine-tenths closed, focus at the tip of the nose. After a while, you will feel a tremendous lead-like sensation in the frontal lobe. The frontal lobe of the brain controls your personality. After a long period of daily practice, the sensation will be lighter, and you will strengthen your elementary personality. When your eyes are focused on the tip of the nose, the mind becomes locked. It cannot move. It is called *Trikutri drishti*. Therefore learn to consolidate and bring your mind to rest. Every individual has a unit of fact of strength within himself to the polarity of the magnetic field. His system is automatic and voluntarily controlled. Indeed, your one and only power is your own mind. In the blink of an eye, it can deliver you to God or the devil; make you bright or depressed. You have to know how your mind works, and then make friends with it. Otherwise, it will run over you.

Let's examine the mind's components. The brain possesses a hypothalamus, a frontal lobe, and a stem. We have three nervous systems. They are all controlled by the motor system in the back of the brain. We have a brain stem, which controls our biological, physical and endurance qualities. Then we have gray matter and neurons which work and pattern our strength, out totality, including how to penetrate through things and what to do. This is called our desiring center. Our frontal lobe is where we think, imagine and see through for strength. The hypothalamus is right on the upper palate. God lives on the tip of the tongue of the saint and the sage. Happiness lives on the tip of the tongue of the human.

Therefore, the tip of your tongue is a precious thing. Try to understand what you are going to create when you use it. The most powerful instrument in our body is the tongue. It has no bones. It can destroy your entire life, or raise you to the pinnacle of success. It is one little piece of meat in the mouth. It can do everything. It can destroy or make you. It is very intelligent. It lives within thirty-two solid teeth. Thirty-two eating animals around it. When your tongue comes up, you are dead. It is a very unique and powerful thing. It can give you what nothing else can give you.

By causing your tongue to move in a permutation and combination, touching the upper palate where there are meridian points for the hypothalamus, it can totally change the neurons of the brain, organize your system to your own capacity and give you that solid divinity which you need. It can also give you intuition. By stimulating the upper palate, the hypothalamus helps the gray matter make the patterned neurons. Once a pattern is completed, God is found.

Feeling shaky can happen to us many times in life. At that time, we can use all of our energy to cover ourselves. One simple method to do this is to inhale deeply, turn your tongue and press it against the palate, then exhale. Inhale and repeat. Just do it subtly so that other people may not know what you are doing. Press your palate again and let it go.

If the breath is reduced to ten times per minute, you can face any challenge. Your life, the force within you, is the breath of life. The average breath rate is fifteen times per minute. If your breath comes up to twenty times per minute, you will be a nervous wreck. You will not be able to think. The stem of the brain will send all the energy to your glandular system just to keep you alive. The stem of the brain plays the most important part in the human mechanism. No matter how stuck you are, breathe mechanically, deeply and consciously and lock it with the hypothalamus. Your own brain pattern will give you the cue of how to resolve the problem on the spot.

In addition, the mind has three primary chambers: negative, positive, and neutral, as well as eighty-one parts. Together, the three primary chambers and eighty-one parts create eighty-four facets, each of which relates to those aspects that create totality of mind. Now, the brain has the very difficult task of calculating its eighty-four aspects along with the seventy-two facets of life in one trillionth of a second. In other words, in any given situation, your mind is capable of seventy thousand projections and has the capacity to calculate thirty trillion megacycles per one zero point of a second. (Interestingly, we also have seventy thousand nerve centers in our feet.) This is super fast. Our memory has its own motor system, projection, and intuition. Within the facets of the mind is the capacity to know yesterday and today, while imagining tomorrow. But, to escape from the guessing game of life, our mind must possess intuitive value. Without intuition, it is impossible to know what the future may bring and we will be extremely insecure. When our control center, which is our mind, errs and does not send the appropriate reinforcements to our cells, we experience disease and unfortunate adjustments in our level of prosperity and social life. Things simply go wrong.

As our spiritual teacher and protector, the third eye relates to knowledge, wisdom, and the development of intuition. It sees what our other two eyes cannot. One of our primary goals is to open the conscious third eye in order to accurately see what it is we need to do, receive, extend, contract, and expel. By the power of the Word, we are given the golden key that opens this heavenly doorway between the eyebrows. For, directly behind the eyebrows lies the pituitary gland, which is the seat of our third eye. It is the realm of projected truth, which is divine, infinite and safe, and the arena of projection and sophistication. There are eighty-four pressure points, and two rows of meridian points, on the upper palate of the human mouth. When you chant the Word, the tongue hits these points, stimulating the hypothalamus which, in turn, makes the pineal gland radiate. When the pineal gland radiates, it creates an impulsation in the pituitary. The entire glandular system then secretes and the individual attains bliss. Cultivating the ability to concentrate deeply at the third eye point, while calmly willing something into being, is what causes the object of your willing to manifest. This is due to the fact that, at the same time that your will is being activated, your meditative mind is being accessed. Moreover, when we meditate on the third eye, we stimulate the central nervous system, which is the operation of the solar, lunar, and neutral currents.

It is within the divine gland and especially the third eye—the Christ center and the location of the pituitary gland—that true happiness is found. The spiritual eye is the entryway into the ultimate state of divine consciousness. In deep meditation, as one's consciousness penetrates the spiritual eye, he successively experiences the following states: superconsciousness, or the ever new joy of soul realization, and oneness with God, or the Holy Ghost; Christ consciousness, oneness with the universal intelligence of God in all creation; Cosmic Consciousness, unity with the omnipresence of God that is beyond, as well as within, vibratory manifestation. Through his divine eye, the yogi steers his consciousness into omnipresence and fills his body with light. Those who master and vibrate at the sixth spiritual center are released from problems as duality dissolves and unity is established in the consciousness. It is here that we meditate on our true nature by connecting with the internal voice of God. We speak consciously because we are aware of the far-reaching effects of our words. We gain psychic powers and destroy all karma we have incurred in past lives. Mastery of this center brings the knowledge that spiritual devotion is the only sure path to liberation. Your spiritual eye is your single eye of intuition and omnipresent perception at the Christ center between the eyebrows. For instance, one can behold the spiritual eye in a ring of golden light encircling a sphere of opalescent blue, and at the center, a pentagonal white star.

Microcosmically, these forms and colors epitomize respectively, the vibratory realm of creation known as cosmic Nature, or Holy Ghost, the son or intelligence of God in creation known as Christ Consciousness, and the vibrationless Spirit beyond all creation known as God, the Father.

Intuition is best described as an inner capability, a latent potential to raise the consciousness of the mind so that the perceptive ability of the individual shifts, and he is able to accurately perceive the truth beyond the illusion of reality. It is the powerful voice of the soul that tells us when something is working or not, and when someone is well meaning or not. Intuition is the force that opens us to receive knowledge from a plane of higher spiritual truths. It is the all-knowing faculty of the soul that enables man to experience direct perception of truth without the intermediary of the senses. The scriptures say this: *O man, go and lie flat at the feet of anyone who can show you how to relate to the unseen.* The third eye doesn't see the seen, but the unseen from whence we came and to where we will return. When our intuition is fully active, we find the answers to the mysteries of the universe.

The heart too, holds a hidden and wonderful divine power. This sacred power can be developed and nurtured by maintaining a universal attitude. A universal attitude secures success in both the material and spiritual worlds. In this age of spirit, it is invaluable, for it shortens the path that leads to the higher spiritual spheres. Practicing with the Word aids in developing and maintaining a universal attitude, while granting the personal magnetism that creates beauty and attracts others. It is both soothing and healing to the practitioner as well as to those with whom he comes into contact. Above all, practicing with the Word can lead us to the desired path of service.

The Word will help you realize that we are all interconnected. Indeed, we are all interconnected throughout the universe. We often act as if we are separate from one another; in fact, we are representations of a greater whole, a manifestation of a law of the universe that binds us to one another. When we pray, we ask to be connected to the Creator and his universal plan, linking us in harmony to all other living beings. We must take the time to connect with our hearts and pray for the world so as to create a greater platform for peace and healing in the world. Let us pray, because prayer is the breathing of the soul which brings help from Heaven. Let us pray so we may all go in this process in the name of God. Anything done in the name of God brings blessings. It is at the beginning of an action that we must pray in order to be sure to embark on the best path with the best forces, so that everything may come back as blessings on ourselves and on others. Let us merge with the light of our hearts, for light is the symbol of all that is purest, most powerful, most beautiful and most sublime. Therefore, let us pray during these complex times so that we may receive blessings from Heaven and gracefully face the challenges of our personal and collective destiny. Let us pray for all, for ourselves and for the world. We must pray so as to dwell in the shelter of Heaven, so we may rest in the shadow of the Luminous Beings and feel our connection to them. Prayer is the power that all human beings have by birthright; when we speak the Word, the Luminous Beings from the invisible world come to our service in the physical world. We must also keep in mind that if every prayer were answered, we would have more misery, more inconvenience, and more trouble than currently exists; therefore, pray wisely, and for the best interest of all. Prayer is the simplest act, its impact seems invisible, yet it can accomplish everything. It is the heavenly power that transforms all misfortune into delight, because it is a godly act from the heart. Blessed is the man or woman who practices with the Word and makes the Lord their trust. Those who pray shall inherit the land of light, and shall delight in the abundance of peace.

*Our hands are our most powerful spiritual
friends and helpers we have.
By working with the forces hidden in our hands,
everything within us becomes organized and harmonious.
The hands allow us to introduce the balance
and harmony of the cosmic into our lives.*

1

THE HIDDEN FORCES IN OUR HANDS

THE TWO GREAT MYSTERIES OF THE UNIVERSE lie in the ineffable power of the Word and the beauty of the hands. True spiritual evolution requires understanding and skillful implementation of the Word and hand symbols. Naam Yoga is the discipline and practice that grants us such knowledge. Naam and hand symbols are the ways in which we communicate with the invisible world, and the most potent tools we have in achieving health, harmony and balance. Indeed, proper use of Naam and the hands, through healing mudras, can alter the course of destructive energies.

Our hands are a beautiful reflection of the universe in which God dwells. God impregnated human hands with His essence, thereby making them a symbolic representation of the life that flows through the totality of creation. The hands, then, are magical instruments, for they contain all principles, the three Gunas, the five elements, the seven spiritual centers, and all factors God employed in order to create the material world. The superiority of man, therefore, lies in and is owed to his hands. As the active agent of the passive powers of the entire system, the hands are the organs of organs. Their beautiful, spiritual forces are ready to aid you when called upon, and they serve as the swords that protect your aura. The science of the hands is powerful in its ability to help you blossom into your highest potential.

Together, the hands function like antennae in that they are able to pick up and project currents of energy. Masters know how to use their hands to receive or project forces, restrain or direct forces, and increase or decrease forces. Significant is the fact that we have ten fingers, for this design links the hands to the cosmic powers of the ten Sephiroth of the Tree of Life. All of our ten fingers correspond to the ten regions of the universe which Kabbalists refer to as Sephiroth. Each single Sephirah is identified by five names which are symbolized by the five fingers on each hand. Those five names are: The name of God, the name of the Sephirah, the name of the leader of the Angelic order of the given Sephirah, the name of the Angelic order, and finally, the name of the planet that rules the Sephirah. There is a tremendous power in our hands and that power is far greater when a human being uses them to work with the Sunlight fluid. These ten Sephiroth are the basis of the two tables of laws Moses placed in the Ark of the Covenant. Moses worked miracles through the ten Sephiroth. Ten represents the fullness of the being, and thanks to our ten fingers all is possible. One must never underestimate the gift of the ten fingers. They are of great value. Again, they are the outward manifestation of the ten Sephiroth that lay within. In other words, our hands are miniature trees of life, impregnated with forces so harmonious and beneficial that their leaves heal every illness and their fruit bestows eternal life. When the forces of the hands are used to attach the miniature tree with the parent tree, immortality is achieved.

Proper use of the hands opens the doors of the higher worlds, allowing you to enjoy the delights therein. Each hand, in and of itself, is a region inhabited by a hierarchy of luminous spirits governed by an Archangel who is, in turn, subject to God. Therefore, it is God Himself who ultimately rules over each of the ten fingers. Understand that even as God is One, His expression changes and He manifests differently according to the given finger. When you wish to enter into one of the angelic regions governed by God, all you need to do is use your hands. Two things are necessary if the hands are to be used in the manner outlined. Firstly, one must learn about the mysterious ways of the hands. Our sacred wisdom is essential here, as it contains a wealth of knowledge concerning the human hands and their power. Secondly, one must become a true yogi and Kabbalist who works solely with the forces of light.

One must consider that the hands are an extension of the heart, which is located in the chest and is the seat of our magnetic field. The chest gives birth to life, and then preserves it. The heart, that center of corporeal form that pumps the life-blood through the body, is the seat of man's animal life as well as his affections, emotions, and sentiments. As such, it is the altar upon which man must offer daily fragrances to his divinity, and maintain the sacred fire that burns all sacrifices. Because of its location in the chest, the heart has higher interests that exert a more refined influence on the individual than those of his stomach and appetites.

One must also consider the intimate connection between the hands and the brain. While the hands are the most amazing of instruments, they require the direction of the brain. Indeed, all that is performed by the hands is first commanded by the brain, that seat of mind and intelligence located at a considerable distance from the hands themselves. As the hands are dependent on the brain for their intelligence, they naturally reflect the type of brain that guides them.

The ancient yogis mapped out certain areas on the hands and their associated reflexes. When you understand this coding, you understand that the hands are an energy map of our consciousness and health. Every part of your body and brain can be accessed and stimulated through a corresponding part of your hand(s). The hands contain more nerves than any other part of the human system, with the greatest concentration in the palms. The nerves that reach from the brain to the hands are so highly developed due to generational use that they have rendered the hands, whether passive or active, the immediate servant of the brain which is located in your head. The head gives birth to thought, which it manifests. It is upon thought that we depend for our understanding of the mystery of the triad of Nature, Human, and God, as well as of the character of the absolute omneity. In the head of man, his intelligence is found. The role of this intelligence is to control and direct all lower faculties according to their particular laws. Of note is the fact that, according to medical research, a nerve is, in reality, two nerve chords in one sheath. One conveys the action from the brain to the receiving part, and the other conveys the action of the receiving part to the brain. Nerve communication is, therefore, a two way street. Because so many nerves reside in the hands, they have direct communication with every portion of the brain. This makes it possible for them to reveal those portions, or qualities, that are active, those that are dormant, and those that will eventually be developed.

The art of connecting with the forces hidden in our hands is a powerful spiritual cure that brings balance to our energy flow, while restoring and recharging the divine protective shield around us. Use your hands to connect with heaven, and the heavenly life will flow in and around you to produce a life that is lived with the maximum light, effectiveness, and humility. Use your hands to harmonize your vibration with heaven, so that the forces of nature can hear and understand you. Use your hands and go within to consciously experience your beauty as an extension of God. Know that man, in his essence, is infinite, unlimited creative power. When you work with your hands in the attitude of humility and service, their forces will illuminate and immortalize your body, making it divine. Connecting with the powerhouse that is the higher world is the key. By using the hands we can attract luminous beings and cause them to assist us. Hands can be used to create love and harmony. To be a true child of God, one must know how to stretch out one's hands to receive forces from above and project them onto one's self and others in order to restore, balance and cleanse, heal and give life. The hands are a very potent spiritual instrument.

If you want your inner lamp to brighten beyond measure, you must use your hands to plug into the power line above. Understand, however, that the community of light only opens the doors of its school to those who operate with love in the spirit of service and humility. Love solves all problems, and without it we are left with emptiness.

Each of your two hands is home to five unequal fingers that represent various aspects of existence. For example, each finger stands for one of the five elements. Beginning with the thumb and ending with the pinkie, these elements are: earth, water, fire, air, and ether.* By these five elements we live and die and are born again; these are the basis of our

---

* In another school of thought, the elements from the thumb to the pinkie are: fire, air, ether, earth, and water.

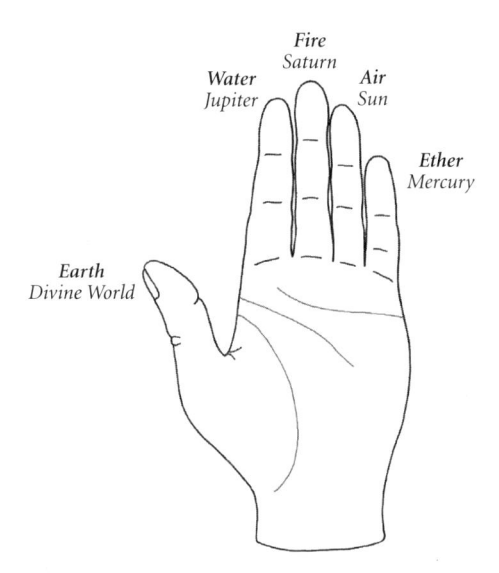

Fire
Saturn
Water
Jupiter
Air
Sun
Ether
Mercury
Earth
Divine World

world and being, and from them all wisdom can be plucked like ripe fruit for the eating. That is why the hand is a symbol which represents the occult maxim "as above so below". We have to use our hands in order to bring forth the wisdom of the Divine and spread it here on earth.

Our hands are a symbol of the Sun. For the Sun is the leading star of our solar system, and our hands, much more than our feet, are shaped like a star when we open them widely. A star is often represented by five branches which is the symbol of a human stretched in a circle. The fingers are an extension of our chest or middle body. The middle finger is the longest, and it is called the Saturn finger. It divides the hand down the center. This finger represents the balancing element in our lives. One should not wear a ring on the middle finger because there is already an invisible one there. If one decides to wear a ring on this finger, it must be with an amethyst or a deep blue sapphire to deflect the negative influence of Saturn. Otherwise, those who wear a ring on the Saturn finger without observing these rules, often suffer from anxiety, depression and fear. Another thing is the presence of a star, or a cross at the base or mount of this finger, indicates serious challenges or hard luck. If that is the case, one should bring *Triple Mantra* into one's spiritual practice to protect oneself.

To one side of the Saturn finger is the index finger, known as the Jupiter finger, and the thumb, which represents our will. To achieve concrete realization on the material plane, one often calls upon the qualities found in these three fingers.

On the other side of the Saturn finger lies the ring finger, or the Sun finger, and the pinkie, or Mercury finger. Artistic and scientific discoveries are often the result of the qualities found in these fingers. People who have a ring encircling the base or mount of the Saturn finger have magical and occult powers. Taken individually, the forefinger represents the human spirit and good understanding, the middle finger stands for the human soul, the ring finger the human intellect, and the pinkie finger the human heart.

The thumb is the only digit that, by virtue of its position on the hand, has the power to point or stand upright independent of the other four fingers. It represents good sense and is the digit where the Divine World expresses itself. In Christianity, the thumb represents God. The first finger represents Christ, which means the indicator of the will of God. The second finger represents the Holy Ghost, and is the attendant of the first. Together, these three digits, the thumb, index finger, and middle finger, represent the Trinity.

Our thumb expresses the world of love, the Divine World. The thumb itself is representative of the four fingers. In order for the four fingers to manifest, they need divine help, which is symbolized by the thumb. The intellect and heart of man must receive the support of the Divine World or universal love. So when you have a need for light, warmth or energy, in order to act right and fulfill your task, softly, with a concentrated and confident spirit, put the tip of your thumb to the tips of the other four fingers and say to yourself, in a loving manner, *"I will fulfill God's will, with all my strength, with all my spirit, and with all my heart."* You may also say, *"By the power of the Christ of God within me, who I serve with all my strength, with all my spirit, with all my heart, I will fulfill the will of God, with all my strength, all my spirit and all my heart."*

The thumb, which represents the will, is connected to the center of the brain. Much can be determined by examining the ways in which a newborn displays and uses his fingers. If, some days after birth, he is inclined to keep his thumb inside his fingers, great physical delicacy has been foreshadowed. If the thumb remains inside the fingers seven days after birth the child will be mentally delicate into adulthood. Take a look, and you will notice that people who are mentally weak have very weak thumbs. Moreover, as it is the thumb that is the individualizing force, adults who talk with their fingers covering their thumbs are demonstrating that they have little self-confidence and self-reliance. It is very important to be careful of those bearing short, weak thumbs. Conversely, a good, strong thumb shows that its owner is evolved. This is an individual who will apply their intellectual will, rather than brute force, to accomplish their desires.

It took the most luminous and superior heavenly beings to work very hard in order to create our hands. Keep your hands clean by washing them when you think they are dirty, so as to maintain the purity of what they represent.

The fingers are the masterful work of the heavenly, the elevated, and the angelic. Many powerful heavenly beings have worked very hard to create the forefinger, which is the finger of the old God of Jupiter called Zeus. It also took numerous elevated beings from the higher world to create the middle finger, a finger of consciousness and justice. It took a tremendous number of angels of high intellect to create the third finger of the Sun that shows a tendency toward that which is beautiful, such as art, music, science, and poetry. It took several angels of good hearts to create the pinkie finger, which is the finger of Mercury, the messenger of the Gods. Having been given these gifts that are our fingers and hands, we must learn to work with them so that they are able to help us remove our weaknesses and receive strength from the higher world. The truth is that our brains, our emotions, and our behaviors can all be therapeutically affected by working correctly with their corresponding areas of the hands.

It is possible to communicate with the mind and body via the sacred sign language of the fingers. This language includes various actions such as curling, crossing, stretching, and touching the fingers and their tips together. In this instance, the hands become the keyboard, the fingers the keys, which serve the mind and body. Touching the tip of the index finger, which represents Jupiter—the planet of expansion—with the tip of the thumb creates *Gyan Mudra*. This mudra bestows receptivity and calmness. When involved in active exercises, the yogi can use a form of this mudra whereby the index finger is bent under the thumb so that its fingernail rests on the thumb's second joint. The attitudes and postures adopted during mudra practices establish a direct link between the physical body, the mental body and the pranic body, and help develop awareness of the flow of prana throughout the entire system. Mudras facilitate pranic balance and redirect the subtle energy into the higher chakras, inducing higher states of consciousness. If you wear pure white and meditate on certain sound currents along with specific mudras for two and half hours a day for one year, you will know the unknowable and see the unseen. Through this constant practice, the mind awakens to the infinite capacity of the soul for sacrifice, service, and creation.

MUDRAS: HAND SEALS

Our hands are our most powerful spiritual friends and helpers we have. By working with the forces hidden in your hands, everything within you will become organized and harmonious. They will allow you to introduce the balance and harmony of the cosmic into your life. Every time you need help you can do a particular mudra and develop the qualities of energies it contains. Whatever you need, whether it be light, love and strength, protection, justice of life, look for it in your hands. You will find that they bring order and balance in your life. Concentrate on a particular mudra for sometime, and try to nurture and strengthen its energies in you. The term mudra refers to the manner in which the hands and fingers are positioned during the practice of chanting mantra. Thousands of mudras exist. Choosing the appropriate mudra and executing it properly can bring about miraculous improvements in the human body. Mudras are known to bring about a quick and fundamental reversal of destructive physical processes such as memory loss, arthritis, gastric difficulties, insomnia, heart disease, abnormal blood pressure, and incurable infections. Moreover, mudras aid in smoothing out character defects by helping to develop the virtuous, sociable, non-violent, pious, and polite aspects of one's disposition. Ultimately, mudras work because they awaken the cosmic energy within and help you merge with the consciousness of the Supreme Soul.

Mudras, the yogic infusions that help to purify the body, can create a healthy level of elements in the body. You can decrease or slow down the level of the elements in the body to calm the turmoil and cool off the fire. This is significant, as it is when the elements are at the highest level of normalcy, that the mind, body, and spirit achieve a state of health and can be devoted to a higher order. Regular application of mudras grants internal strength. Indeed, all Godly and superhuman individuals would remain in mudras for quite a long time. The length of time needed to increase and stabilize the body's elements varies according to the mudra. Some mudras do the work within a few seconds, some within three minutes, and others within 31 to 62 minutes. By the practice of mudra, the elements in the body can be increased and stabilized. This can be done by touching the thumb to the tip of the fingers. Each element may be decreased by bending any finger on the mount of Venus (the pad of flesh at the base of the thumb) and touching the base of the thumb with the tip of the finger.

The practice of mudra is both a science and an art. Meditations with mudras are very precise in terms of the reaction they produce in the body and psyche through specific coded action, and artistic in the way they mold consciousness and refine sensation and insight. Hand gestures are spiritual, emotional, and devotional gestures or attitudes. A mudra is an attitude of energy flow, intended to link our individual pranic force with the universal or cosmic force.

Hand seals create circuits that combine subtle physical movements which alter mood, attitude, and physical perception, and deepen awareness and concentration. A mudra may be a simple hand position or involve the whole body in a combination of posture, breath, locks and visualization techniques. Mudras are used in higher practices of consciousness, which lead to the awakening of the pranas, chakras, and kundalini, and which can bestow major *siddhis* (spiritual mastery) and psychic powers upon the advanced practitioner. Mudras manipulate prana in much the same way that energy in the form of light or sound waves is diverted by a mirror or a cliff face. The nadis and chakras constantly radiate prana which normally escapes from the body and dissipates into the external world. By creating barriers within the body through the practice of mudra, the energy is redirected within. Mudras are especially important techniques in awakening kundalini, due to their ability to redirect prana. Scientifically, mudras influence the unconscious reflexes and primal, instinctive habit patterns that originate in the primitive area of the brain stem by establishing a subtle, non-intellectual connection with these areas. Each mudra sets up a different link and has a correspondingly different effect on the body, mind and prana. The goal is to create repetitive postures and gestures which interrupt the circuit of habitual, instinctive patterns and establish a more refined consciousness.

Gyan Mudra

Gyan Mudra and Chin Mudra are psycho-neural finger locks which make meditation work more powerfully. The palm and fingers of the hand have many nerve root endings which constantly emit energy. When the finger touches the thumb, a circuit is produced which allows the energy that would normally dissipate into the environment to travel back into the body and up the brain. The fingers and hands are placed on the knees, thus sensitizing the knees and creating another pranic circuit that maintains and redirects prana within the body. In addition, placing the hands on the knees stimulates a nadi which runs from the knees up the inside of the thighs and into the perineum. This nadi is known as *Gupta*, or hidden nadi. Sensitizing this nadi helps stimulate the energy at the first chakra. When the palms are placed upward in Chin Mudra the chest area opens up. The practitioner may experience a sense of lightness and receptivity which is otherwise absent during the practice of Gyan Mudra with the palms facing down. The index finger represents the air element. Traditionally, it is folded down into the mount of Venus to decrease the level of air, which is mental activity.

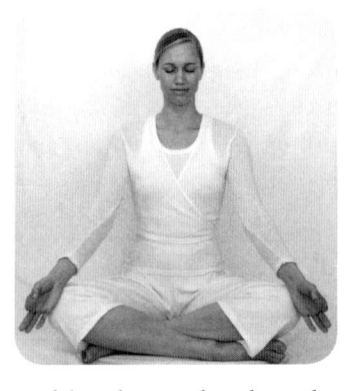

The effect of Gyan and Chin Mudra is very subtle, and it requires great sensitivity on one's part to perceive the change in consciousness. This sensitivity is established and strengthened through practice. *Gyana* means wisdom or knowledge; thus, Gyan Mudra is a gesture of intuitive knowledge. *Chin*, which is derived from the chit, or chitta, means consciousness; thus, this mudra is the psychic gesture of consciousness. Symbolically, the pinkie, ring, and middle fingers represent the three *Gunas* or qualities of nature: *tamas*, or inertia; *rajas*, or activity and creativity; and *sattva*, or luminosity and harmony. In order for consciousness to pass from ignorance to knowledge, these three states must be transcended. Also, it is important to note that the index finger represents individual consciousness, the *jiv atma*, while the thumb represents supreme consciousness. In Gyan and Chin Mudra, the individual (index finger) is bowing down to the supreme consciousness (the thumb), acknowledging its unsurpassed power. The index finger however is touching the thumb, symbolizing the ultimate unity of the two experiences and the culmination of yoga.

Gyan Mudra is known as the "Mother of Great Knowledge." Benefits of this mudra include high levels of concentration, which connect you to joy and awareness, greater balance for mentally disturbed or agitated people, and a magnification of mental powers, while the pulse readjusts to a healing rhythm. A consistent practice will bestow a beautiful aura and healing influence for others. This mudra is also beneficial for mental depression and drug addiction, changing a hard nature and a cold heart to a charming, cordial nature while divine knowledge and Godly vision takes firm hold within the soul. Gyan Mudra has numerous benefits. It strengthens all the tendons and veins throughout the body, and gives the practitioner great mental power, along with improved memory. Another beneficial effect of the mudra is that it slowly cures insomnia by creating healing conditions in the minute sensory nerve cells of the brain. The mudra automatically cures numerous mental ailments, bad habits, addictions to intoxicants or drugs. It will turn a non-believer into a believer, restoring faith in the universe to those in despair.

Gyan Mudra fills you with spiritual thoughts and desires to be committed to your work, duties and responsibilities; you develop a true capacity to serve. When you practice this mudra, you can live in the material world, performing all your duties, and still remain detached from material reality as your inner eyes open and you begin to experience real enlightenment. This mudra destroys depression and lack of interest in life, removing half-heartedness and indecision from your consciousness. It brings freedom from vanity and worldly desires; ignorance disappears, and true contemplation is possible. One reaches the threshold of divine knowledge. This divine science of the supreme self, coupled with the understanding of astronomy and how the planets affect the universe, will permit you to access the greatest storehouse of healing, which is available to all. By practicing with this mudra one can control the mind, which is the restorer of all the organs. It will help you to enjoy life while still experiencing a feeling of detachment from worldly concerns, because it removes the internal darkness caused by vanity and greed. This mudra will move you to the level of a yogi and Kabbalist of the highest order, so that you may enjoy the indescribable exhilaration of living as a supreme soul. Through dedication to this mudra, every question of your mind, heart and soul will be answered, and many other secrets of the world will be revealed. As you receive this Divine Spiritual Wisdom, you will release negative mental habits, which will brighten your soul and put a glow on your face.

Those who practice this mudra will experience profound changes in their minds and hearts. Consistent practice of the mudra will assist the gray matter of the brain to experience beneficial changes. You become fearless, bold, and courageous, even to the point where you do not fear the angel of death. This mudra also alleviates anxiety and gives you stamina to face life's problems. You will acquire wisdom and knowledge, as well as detachment. This mudra cures ailments associated with the tissue that encircles the ligaments. With Gyan Mudra, one gains the experience and capacity to go into deep meditative consciousness. Use these mantric experiences to fully explore the infinity at the center of neutrality.

Most hand mudras are meditative seals used to redirect the prana that is emitted by the hands back into the body. Mudras which join the thumb and index finger engage the motor cortex at a very subtle level, generating a loop of energy which moves from the brain down the hand

and then back again. Conscious awareness of the process rapidly leads to internalization and enlightenment.

Most people have learned that there are two versions of Gyan Mudra, but there are many subtle variations.

Gyan Mudra is called the spiritual gesture of knowledge. Traditionally, the index finger curls into the inside root of the thumb, and the other fingers remain straight and slightly apart. Hands are resting on the knees with the palms facing down. The hands and the arms are relaxed.

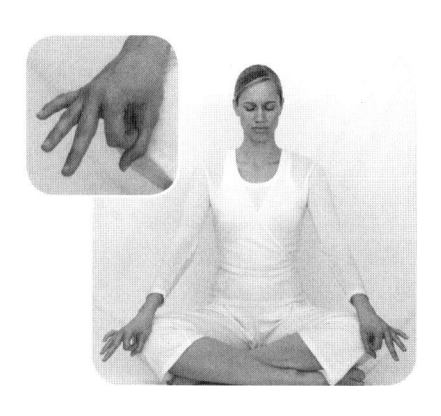

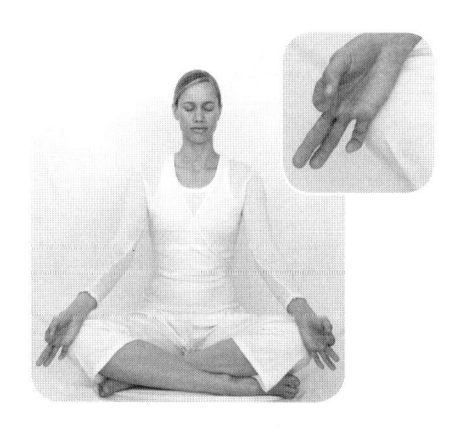

Chin Mudra is a version of Gyan Mudra. It is called a spiritual gesture of consciousness. According to tradition, the index finger is also folded into the root of the thumb with the hands resting on the knees, but in this version the palms face up to open the chest to allow for deep breathing.

Active Gyan Mudra is performed with the thumb pressed over the fingernail of the index finger, palm facing up. This helps impart knowledge, expansion and spirituality.

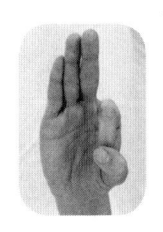

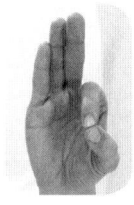

Passive (or Divine) Gyan Mudra is performed with the thumb tip pressed to the index fingertip, palm facing up. When the tip of the index finger meets the thumb—when man meets God—it removes aggression and brings calmness and peace of mind.

For Wisdom and to Override the Ego: This particular Gyan Mudra is not only for wisdom, it also helps one override the ego. Here, the thumb tip is pressed in the crook between the first and second phalanges* of the index finger.

Grounding Gyan Mudra is used ground yourself. The index fingertip is pressed to the crook of the thumb between the first and second phalanges; the hands face down.

For Muscular Ailments, Rheumatism, and Sciatica: When the Jupiter finger placed on the mount of Venus (the pad of flesh at the base of the thumb) with the thumb tip over the middle knuckle of the index finger, it stops muscular ailments, rheumatism and sciatica.

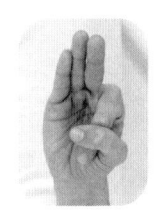

*Note: Each finger has three phalanges or sections: the first phalange is the section with the fingernail; the next is the second phalange, and third phalange is adjacent to the palm.

Shuni Mudra

Touch the tip of the middle finger to the tip of the thumb, and you have Shuni Mudra. This mudra grants discipline, patience and discernment, as the middle finger symbolizes the planet Saturn—the Lord of Karma who makes us muster the courage we need to live up to our responsibilities.

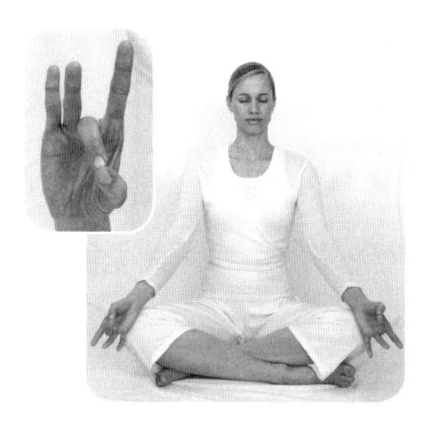

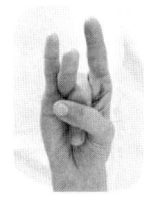

Saturn on the Venus mount: This is performed by placing the tip of the middle (Saturn finger) on the Venus mount, which is the pad of flesh on the palms at the base of the thumb, and lock it with your thumb. This mudra helps ear ailments and also nose and throat.

Surya or Ravi Mudra

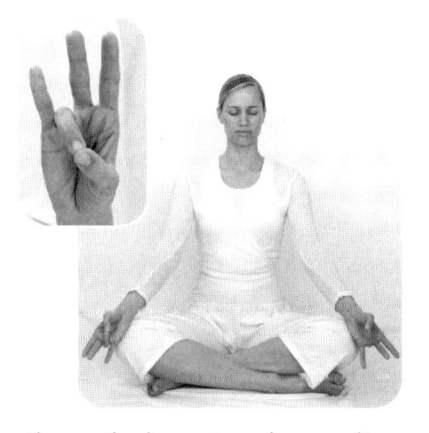

Place the tip of the ring finger on the tip of the thumb, and you have Surya or Ravi Mudra. The ring or Sun finger is your radiant body. It is your brightness, your shield. Working with this mudra bestows revitalizing energy, nervous strength, and good health. The prolonged practice of this posture removes vitamin deficiencies, especially those created by the earth element, and normalizes the natural equilibrium of the body. Repetition increases the glow, or luster of the body, imparting goodness and transcendental spiritual qualities. One moves from narrow mindedness to broad mindedness and compassion. Practicing the mudra will encourage the natural flow of happiness throughout the body, bringing joy, vigor and vitality to every cell. Tolerance and patience will flood your being, and your thought processes will be filled with benevolence and desire for stability. The ring finger symbolizes the Sun or Uranus. The Sun represents energy, health, and sexuality. Uranus represents nervous strength, intuition, and change. Ravi Mudra increases general immunity to disease. It builds the nerve strength and rebalances the electromagnetic field of the body.

Buddhi Mudra

With the tip of the little finger on the tip of the thumb, you have Buddhi Mudra. The pinkie or Mercury finger is your word. One wrong word and you are all wrong. One right word and you are all right. With the use of your words, you can create havoc for yourself, or you can create heaven in your life. Working with this mudra opens one's capacity to communicate clearly and intuitively.

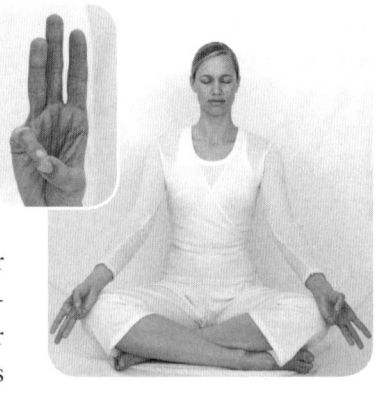

Working with this finger can help take care of the healthy level of water in your body. It is important to normalize the water element in the body so that you may cure many diseases and illnesses caused by an internal decrease of water. Over sixty-percent of the body is composed of water; when this percentage decreases, the body tightens and feels uncomfortable and sore. Certain medications cause the balance of water in the body to become threatened, polluting half the blood supply and creating further ailments. This posture removes dryness within the body, healing all ailments connected with dehydration and enhances physical beauty. It also stimulates psychic development. The little finger symbolizes Mercury, the planet of quickness and the mental powers of communication.

THE VARIOUS HEALING TRIANGLES

There are five healing triangles: the Golden Triangle, Silver Triangle, Purifying Triangle, Centering Triangle, and Copper Triangle.

Golden Triangle

As said early the three digits, the thumb, index finger, and middle finger, represent the Trinity. When they come together, they create the Golden Triangle. The Golden Triangle can heal those suffering from high blood pressure in just a few days. Heart problems come from high blood pressure, incorrect eating and drinking habits, excessive worries, lack of sufficient rest, and a lack of peace during the digestive process. The current of air in the veins is the circulation of blood in the body. When it moves very fast the diseases created by the high blood pressure create disturbances in the lungs, arteries and veins. This leads to symptoms such as red eyes, sleeplessness, turmoil, headaches, and other problems throughout the body. This can be corrected by the Golden Triangle.

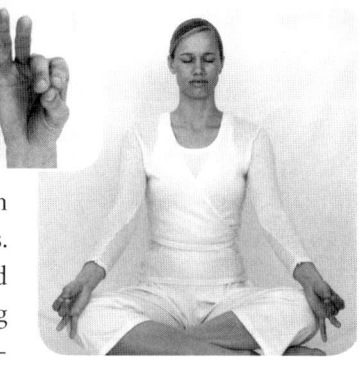

The Golden Triangle is a hand mudra that has been used to access the radiant and healing energy contained in the invisible and mysterious Sunlight fluid within and around us. The thumb symbolizes the three ruling powers of will, logic, and love. The index finger represents Jupiter, the Lord of Prosperity. The middle finger, Saturn, signifies discipline and balance. Jupiter represents the water element, and Saturn represents the fire element. By putting the thumb, Jupiter and Saturn fingers together, the qualities of will, logic and love are used to balance the water and fire elements, thereby steadying these forces in our lives.

Tremendous healing power can be released when a person applies the Golden Triangle to a specific point on their body, or the body of someone who needs healing.

The Golden Triangle can also shape the future according to our desire, as applying it makes it easier to crystallize or manifest wishes.

This mudra is a powerful tool when used in combination with visualization. Try this the next time you are looking for a place to park in the city: Create the Golden Triangle and envision yourself finding a parking space waiting for you. Visualize this with confidence and certitude. By forming the Golden Triangle, you are consolidating your energies and crystallizing your desire in the material plane for a brief moment. You will soon find a parking space.

Here's another example, suppose you are going to an important meeting. Perform the Golden Triangle just before going to sleep. Picture the outcome that you want from the meeting, release the image, and mentally affirm that it is done. Then go to sleep. The outcome will most certainly be positive.

The Golden Triangle can also be used to redirect the invisible Sun light fluid circulating within us to recharge our nervous systems. When you feel your energy is depleted, here's what you can do: *Form the Golden Triangle Mudra and place it exactly at the nape of the neck. Do Breath of Fire (rapid equal inhale and exhale from the diaphragm) for 1 minute or slow and deep breathing for 3 minutes. Then inhale, suspend the breath and think "harmony." Exhale and relax.* You will notice an increase in your energy. This is an excellent quick pick-me-up for the late afternoon lulls.

The reason this works is, the eye of the astral body is located at the nape of the neck, the point where the back of the neck and the head meet. That point is symbolized on the Tree of Life by *Daath*. Daath is our link to another dimension, another reality. Its domain is the throat chakra, which corresponds to the element of ether. The breath is connected with the astral body, and it is the astral body that provides the circulation of this mysterious invisible Sunlight fluid—fluid that is transmuted into the pranic or nervous force within humans. Sleep is also connected with the same astral body, also known as the plastic envelope. During waking hours the nervous force or electricity goes toward the brain for the intellect or consciousness to function. After continuous activity the reserve of the sympathetic nervous system gets used up. At this point, the nervous force changes direction and heads to the spinal matter and sympathetic ganglia. That's when we begin yawning, become tired and sleepy. By using the Golden Triangle at the nape of the neck, and working with the breath, we can restore the nervous force of the astral body and direct a strong current of energy up to the brain, energizing and awakening us.

Here's another way to direct the healing aspect of this invisible Sunlight fluid with the Golden Triangle: *If someone you know has an illness, but doesn't know exactly what it is, have them lie down on their stomach. Form the Golden Triangle and touch the heart center location on their back, between the spine and the left shoulder blade. Feel your mind quiet, calm, and centered, and meditate on the Sun—see and feel its warmth and pure light. Feel that unlimited energy pour from the universe through you to the heart center of the other person. Continue for 3 to 11 minutes.* Remember that you are like a pipe, allowing this mysterious, spiritual, healing force to flow through you to the other person. Improvement will be felt within a few hours.

Silver Triangle

The Silver Triangle is formed by bringing the tips of the thumb, ring and pinkie fingers together. The Silver Triangle Mudra strengthens your energy body and builds your overall power of recuperation. The Silver Triangle Mudra causes sickness to leave and all bad omens fall from the being. With this mudra, all physical ailments will be spiritually healed, and your life will be longer and well-balanced. It energizes the body and improves vitality and eyesight. This mudra is good for those who feel nervous, tired and weak. Remember, it is not you who are doing the healing; it is the grace of the Infinite conscious energy.

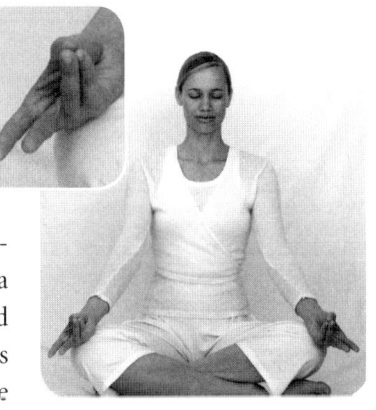

Purifying Triangle

The Purifying (Apana) Triangle is formed by bringing the tips of the thumb, ring and middle fingers together. The ring and pinkie fingers are extended straight. This mudra purifies the body and removes blocks. It provides relief for urinary problems, especially for those who cannot urinate. It also eases difficulty in labor and delivery.

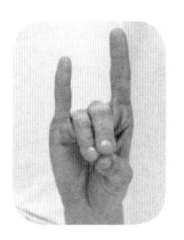

At the moment of birth, before the newborn has uttered his first cry or taken his first breath, his fingers extend with a spasmodic jerk that causes them to rigidly straighten out. It is precisely at this time that the vital spark that sets the human machinery in motion by awakening the mind and habilitating the senses is projected into the child via the extended fingers. Indeed, following the involuntary motion of the hands, the commonly recognized signs of life, a cry, a first breath, take place. Shortly thereafter the child feels hunger, and the hand naturally gravitates to the mouth. From the first moment of life, then, the hands assume their role as a gift from God and the brain's servant.

During the first few months of a child's life, his time is consumed with sleeping, eating, and growing. This growth is demonstrated by the thick development of the first phalanges, which represents the existence of a sensualist whose sole desire is to satisfy his hunger. As the brain unfolds, the mind develops and the child grows. He begins to need less sleep. After the age of eleven, his hands begin to progressively take the shape they will eventually assume. This is the roadmap that will guide him in the future.

Centering Triangle

When you touch the thumb to the Jupiter (index) and Sun (ring) fingers, you create the Centering Triangle Mudra. Activating Sun energy creates balance and strength within the body and nervous system, and pressing on the Jupiter finger enhances the expansive qualities of good health while increasing peace of mind. When you practice this mudra, all dizziness and mental fuzziness disappear. You become grounded and centered.

Copper Triangle
When you touch the thumb to the Saturn (middle) and Mercury (pinkie) fingers, you create the Copper Triangle. This mudra gives relief for a variety of physical difficulties. Touching the Mercury finger activates the energy that resolves problems of the nervous system, including involuntary twitching, nervousness and pinched nerves. Mercury also controls afflictions of the brain and back pain. When you touch the Saturn finger, you are working with issues that directly relate to the bones, liver, intestines and spleen.

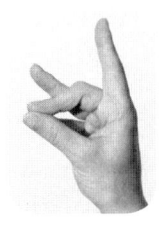

THE FIVE SECRET ROYAL MUDRAS

The Royal Kriya mudras, which work on each of the five fingers, are among the most powerful healing mudras known to humankind. They possess the ability to dramatically improve one's health, for they work to transmute and heal destructive energies stemming from negative emotions. It is these emotions that lead to health problems. Understand that, among other qualities, the five elements—earth, water, fire, air, and ether—indicate the five emotions of worry, fear, anger, joy (excess), and grief. These elements and emotions are represented in the five fingers of each hand. When we work with mudras, we are working on the five elements and five emotions. When one or more are imbalanced and cause health problems, we can choose the Royal Kriya Mudra that highlights the finger representative of the emotional imbalance or health issue. In this way, we can transform the difficulty we may be faced with.

There are many ways in which we can work with the Royal Kriya mudras. If we are experiencing a specific health problem, we want to work with a specific mudra. For example, someone experiencing lung difficulties, such as asthma, would work with the thumb and Raj Kriya Mudra for a total of 30 minutes, as the lung meridian ends in the thumb. If, however, we want to work on our overall health, we need to work with each finger and each Royal Kriya Mudra. Spend 3 minutes on each finger, starting with the left thumb, progressing through the fingers of the left hand, and then the right thumb and fingers. You will cover your ten fingers in 30 minutes, working on your entire body this way.

When we combine the power of the Word with the practice of the Royal Kriya mudras, we call down blessings from God and the universe to help improve every aspect of our health and regain within the precious qualities of hope, love and faith. Working with the Rootlight CDs can accelerate our healing potential. Two mantras have proven to be most beneficial when improving one's state of health through application of the Royal Kriya mudras. The first is *Ra Ma Da Sa Sa Say So Hung* (track 4 on the *The Healing Spirit of RaMaDaSa* CD). The second is *Eck Ong Kar Sat Nam Siri Wahe Guru* (either track on *The Seal of Higher Destiny*). Each of these mantras is approximately 30 minutes in length and can be used in each of the two ways detailed above.

RAJ KRIYA MUDRA *(Thumb/Lungs)*
The lung meridian ends in the thumb. The thumb is connected to the energy of the lungs, which correlates to concerns of the heart. This mudra removes worries. The condition of the thumb and/or thumbnail, then, can be indicative of lung deficiency and/or sadness and troubles of the heart. For example, often times when lung or emotional problems are present there will be a change in nail color, such as a blackening or the appearance of white lines. Other times, the individual will experience pain or the inability to move the thumb. In addition to being associated with the lungs, the human thumb is considered the center of the brain. Indeed, the thumb has its own control section in the brain, which is separate from the other fingers.

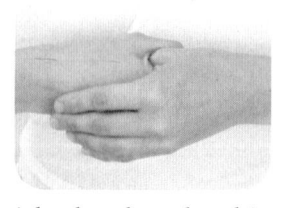

Raj Kriya Mudra is performed by placing the left thumb in the center of the right palm and wrapping the fingers of the right hand around the thumb so that it is enclosed in a loose fist. The fingers of the left hand then come to rest on top of the right. (Note: *Raj Kriya Mudra* can also be performed with the right thumb enclosed in the left hand.) *Raj Kriya Mudra* is used to relieve a variety of emotional and physical difficulties. It energizes the lungs so as to help one avoid and combat asthma, TB, pneumonia and other respiratory diseases. This mudra also revitalizes the brain, bringing order and neutralizing the effects of depression, negativity and worry. With *Raj Kriya Mudra*, the blood is cleansed, the head is cleared, the digestive system is regulated and breathing is improved.

GYAN KRIYA MUDRA *(Index Finger/Large Intestines)*
The large intestine meridian begins at the tip of the index finger. Therefore, pain or numbness, or the inability to bend the index finger without discomfort indicates a dysfunction of the large intestines. In addition, any change in color in the index fingernail is indicative of a large intestine problem.

Gyan Kriya Mudra is performed by placing the left Jupiter (index) finger in the center of the right palm and wrapping the fingers of the right hand around the index finger so that it is enclosed in a loose fist. The fingers of the left hand are held in a relaxed position. (Note: *Gyan Kriya Mudra* can also be performed with the right Jupiter finger enclosed in the left hand.) Problems connected with the large intestine, such as constipation, diarrhea, abdominal pain, irritable bowel syndrome and rectal prolapse, can be treated with the application of *Gyan Kriya Mudra*. Issues linked to the large intestine and Jupiter finger, such as dread and anxiety felt in the pit of the stomach, can also be resolved with *Gyan Kriya Mudra*.

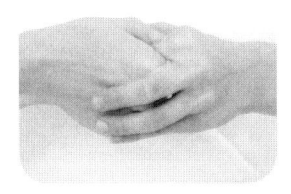

GURU KRIYA MUDRA *(Middle Finger/Pericardium Brain)*
In traditional acupuncture, the pericardium, or membrane around the heart and liver, is considered one of the twelve organs connected with the meridian ending in the middle finger. Recent research states that it also represents the brain and nervous system. Any changes in the middle finger itself or the nail of the middle finger is indicative of a problem in the pericardium or nervous system.

Guru Kriya Mudra is performed by placing the left Saturn (middle) finger in the center of the right palm and wrapping the fingers of the right hand around the middle finger so that it is enclosed in a loose fist. The fingers of the left hand are held in a relaxed position. (Note: *Guru Kriya Mudra* can also be performed with the right Saturn finger enclosed in the left hand.) *Guru Kriya Mudra* can assist with a myriad of chest problems including pain or heaviness in the chest, heavy breathing and heart palpitations. Because the liver is linked to anger, this mudra can also correct imbalances that result from too much anger. To do so, perform *Guru Kriya Mudra* with each hand for three or more minutes. As *Guru Kriya Mudra* removes anger, it will harmonize all ascending and descending currents in the body.

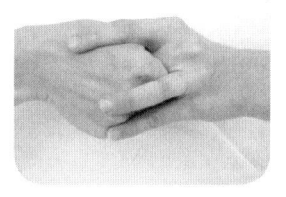

SURYA KRIYA MUDRA *(Ring Finger/Triple Warmer-Spinal Cord)*
The ring, or Sun, finger is connected to the Triple Burner meridian. Triple Burner refers to the division of the torso into the upper, middle and lower sections. The Upper Burner corresponds to the area between the solar plexus and clavicle. Its function is respiration, and its main organs are the lungs and heart-pericardium. The Middle Burner corresponds to the area between the solar plexus and the navel. Its function is digestion and its main organs are the spleen, stomach, liver, and gallbladder. The Lower Burner corresponds to the area between the navel and the pubic bone. Its function is elimination and its main organs are the kidneys, urinary bladder, and lower intestines. These three areas are complementary in function, each supporting the other. The total health of the body depends upon the harmonious interaction of these three functions. The Triple Burner meridian begins at the outer tip of the ring finger and goes along the back of the hand, wrist, forearm and upper arm, until it reaches the shoulder region where it branches off. One branch travels internally into the chest and passes through the pericardium and diaphragm uniting the upper, middle and lower burners. The other branch runs externally up the side of the neck, circles the ear and face, and finally ends at the outer end of the eyebrow where it connects with the gall bladder meridian.

Disharmony in the Triple Burner meridian leads to a whole host of difficulties that manifest in one or more areas of the Triple Burner. Difficulties can include abdominal distention, edema, melancholy, urinary incontinence or difficulty urinating, loss of hearing and tinnitus, as well as pain in the throat, eyes, cheeks, backs of the ears, shoulders, and upper arms. Moreover, the Triple Burner meridian controls the temperature of all organs, as well as their function. When heat is left unchecked in the stomach and spleen, gas, ulcers, hyperacidity, burning, burping, inflammation of the stomach, anemia, sickle cell, leukemia and hemophilia can result. Working with the Triple Burner meridian can treat such disturbances. Any disturbance dealing with fever, such as rheumatic fever, typhoid fever, pneumonia, colds, or flu, can also be cured using this meridian, particularly in children.

Symptoms of the ring finger, such as pain or the inability to bend it, indicate that the Triple Warmer meridian is in trouble and that the individual is susceptible to the difficulties detailed above. To correct the problem(s), work with *Surya Kriya Mudra*. *Surya Kriya Mudra* is performed by placing the left Sun (ring) finger in the center of the right palm and wrapping the fingers of the right hand around the ring finger, so that it is enclosed in a loose fist. The fingers of the left hand are held in a relaxed position. (Note: *Surya Kriya Mudra* can also be performed with the right Sun/ring finger enclosed in the left hand.)

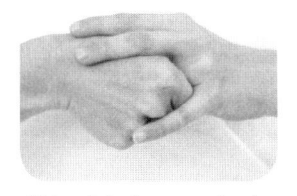

BUDDHI KRIYA MUDRA *(Little Finger/Heart & Small Intestines)*
The Mercury, or little, finger influences our communication, and represents the heart and small intestines. The heart meridian ends in the inner side of the little fingernail and the small intestine meridian starts at the outer side of the nail. Pain in the little finger, or discoloration of the little fingernail, forewarns of heart-related problems or trouble in the small intestines.

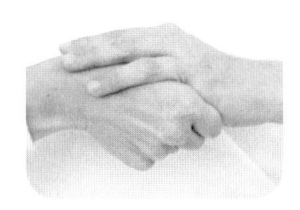

Buddhi Kriya Mudra is performed by placing the left Mercury (little) finger in the center of the right palm and wrapping the fingers of the right hand around the little finger, so that it is enclosed in a loose fist. The fingers of the left hand are held in a relaxed position. (Note: *Buddhi Kriya Mudra* can also be performed with the right Mercury finger enclosed in the left hand.) *Buddhi Kriya Mudra* helps the heart, balances the kidneys, prevents urinary disorders and corrects problems with the ears. Indeed, access the heart energy that ends in the pinkie finger through *Buddhi Kriya Mudra* to prevent all heart ailments, including heart attacks and bypass surgery. Were knowledge of this one mudra and its applications widespread, cardiologists would be jobless and echocardiograms would be rendered obsolete. Sleep issues can also be aided with this mudra, as it soothes the nerves and neutralizes all forms of irritations ranging from the mental to the physical. Good sleep will come after gently pressing the bottom of the little fingernail nineteen times. Since the small intestine meridian starts at this little finger, by activating *Buddhi Kriya Mudra*, lactating mothers will cause proper secretion of milk. Finally, because Mercury deals with communication, *Buddhi Kriya Mudra* helps resolve communication issues and helps us to feel comfortable with exactly who we are. With *Buddhi Kriya Mudra*, we no longer feel the need to give others a false impression.

There are many interconnections in the human body. Each of these interconnections has a meridian point that ends in the fingers and thumb. For example, when we touch the thumb to the Jupiter finger, we combine the lung energy ruled by the thumb with the energy of the large intestine that is controlled by Jupiter. The following are examples:
- *The heart is linked to the small intestines*
- *The lungs are linked to the large intestines*
- *The liver is linked to the gall bladder*
- *The spleen and pancreas are linked to the stomach*
- *The kidneys are linked to the urinary tract*

It is essential that we begin to recognize the subtle yet penetrating power of working with hand mudras in connection with Naam to revitalize and heal the body, as well as relieve emotional distress and blockages generated by long-held, negative beliefs.

OTHER MUDRAS FOR HEALING, MEDITATION AND PRAYER

Heart Mudra

Fold the index finger down onto the Venus mount at the base of the thumb and join the tips of the middle and ring fingers to the tip of the thumb, so they are placed side by side. The little finger remains straight. Place the hands on the knees with the palms facing upwards. Close your eyes and relax the whole body, keeping it motionless. This practice may performed for up to 31 minutes. As you practice, focus your attention on the breath in the chest area. In other words, focus on the heart center.

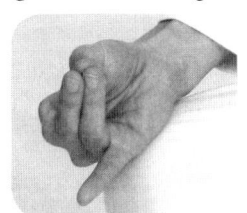

The benefit of this mudra is to divert the flow of prana from the hands to the heart area, improving the vitality of the physical heart. The middle and little fingers relate directly to nadis connected with the heart, while the thumb closes the pranic circuit and acts as an energizer, diverting the flow of prana from the hands to these nadis. This mudra is beneficial for heart ailments, especially ischemic heart in acute situations. The heart is the center of emotion. This mudra helps release pent up emotion and unburdens the heart. It may be practice during emotional conflict and crisis.

Surbhi Mudra

Surbhi Mudra is performed as follows: Touch the Saturn tips to the Jupiter tips, and the Mercury tips to meet the Sun tips. In other words, the index of each hand touches the middle finger of the other. The ring finger of each hand touches the pinkie of the other. All of the fingers are relatively straight and only the tips of each finger touches. The thumbs are straight upward. This mudra is good for students with failing memories; it controls rheumatic inflammation and sharpens the intellect. It is also good for sciatica.

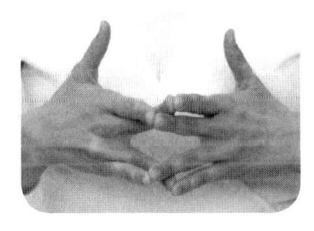

Prayer Pose

Bringing the palms together creates Prayer Pose. In this pose, the positive side of the body (right or male) and negative (left or female) are neutralized. This pose should always be used as you begin your practice, as it centers you in preparation for meditation and works of prayer.

For example, in conjunction with the *Prayer of Love, Peace and Light (page 172),* bring your hands into prayer pose and cross the right thumb over the left thumb. Place the heels of the hands against the sternum or heart level, pointing the hands straight out in front of the body at a 45 degree angle from the chest. Breathe normally and let the breath adjust itself to the meditation. Center the focus and dive deep into the higher realm of existence. Melt the outer self into the inner self. Create a very simple feeling within the mind and just let yourself go. Relax the mind and tell the intellect not to formulate any more thoughts, and focus on the *Prayer of Love, Peace and Light.* By doing the prayer in this posture, it will cause the mudra to neutralize the energy within the body, while you are surrounding yourself and projecting the healing and beneficial vibrations of Love, Peace and Light. Reciting the prayer in this meditation posture has a very soothing effect on the personality. It enables you to meditate on your own divine force, your own fiber. If the fiber of the being is not right, the being itself cannot be right. It is very important to be centered in both focus and hand position. Your capacity as a human being will not give you any upsetting nature if you are centered.

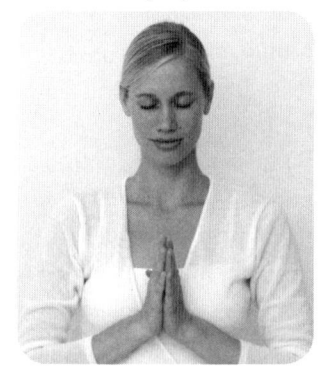

Working with mudras can impart complete mental balance within the individual's psyche. The hand is the blueprint for the electromagnetic field of the aura: the index and ring finger are electrically negative, and the middle and pinkie finger are electrically positive. When you practice Kirtan Kriya (sequentially touching the thumb tip to the index, middle, ring and pinkie fingertips), you alternate your electrical polarities, causing a balance in the electromagnetic projection of the aura.

Venus Lock

Yogis employ the Venus Lock, so named because it connects the positive and negative sides of the Venus mount on each hand to the thumbs. The thumbs represent the ego. The Venus mount is the fleshy area at the base of the thumb. It is symbolic of the planet Venus, which is associated with the energy of sensuality and sexuality. This mudra, then, properly channels sexual energy and promotes glandular balance. It also grants an increased ability to focus easily when resting in your lap while you are in a meditative posture.

To form the mudra, face the palms toward each other. Interlace the fingers with the left thumb tip just above the base of the thumb on the webbing between the right thumb and index finger. The tip of the right thumb presses the fleshy mound near the base of the left thumb. The thumb positions are reversed for women.

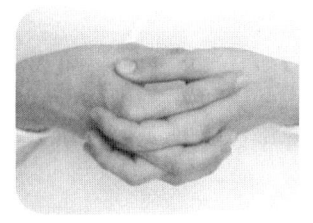

Hands in Lap

Having the hands in the lap is another common mudra for meditation. It is formed by resting the left palm face-up in the lap with the right hand palm-up on top of it. Put the thumb tips together. The hand positions are reversed for women (as shown in the photo).

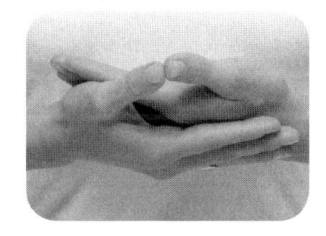

We are all aware that the hands are used as a means of transmission and reception between human beings. The sense of touch, concentrated in the hands especially at the fingertips and center of the palm, is the most indispensable of the five senses. So indispensable is the sense of touch that it can almost act as a replacement for the other four. Think about it for a moment. Those deprived of the ability to see, hear, smell, and taste can all communicate with and navigate the world around them as long as their sense of touch remains unimpaired and their hands are in full possession of their powerful abilities. Even those rendered "dumb" can connect with the world via their hands.

The supremacy of our hands is due to their capacity to absorb and distribute the vital, or astral, fluid in our bodies. The mounts under the four fingers, as well as the hollow of the hand, contain approximately 300 pacinian corpuscles, which are the accumulation of nervous matter. Nerves, then, are richly represented in the hands, not only at the fingertips, where the sense of touch is at its best, but also in the mounts and hollows. Together, the pacinian corpuscles act as the condenser of innervation, allowing the fingertips to receive and store the vital fluid. Stored in the fingertips, this vital fluid becomes a reservoir of electricity that endows the hands with their surprising sensitivity, commonly referred to as the sense of touch. In addition, the poverty or abundance of our vital fluid is visibly reflected on our hands. As the vital, or astral, fluid penetrates our fingertips, accumulates in the pacinian corpuscles, and traces deep channels on the surface of the palm, it eventually reaches the brain. Upon reaching the brain, it is redistributed throughout the body via its innumerable outgrowth of nerves. As the vital fluid in our bodies retraces the path it took to reach the brain, it returns to the ocean that is nature's vital fluid via the fingertips, thereby establishing the connection that allows us to work with currents of energy and natural forces.

There is a vital fluid that permeates certain human organs—the fingers primary among them. It is stored in the cells of the brain, and it surrounds our world and everyone in it. God, the Great Architect of the Universe, created this vital fluid. As we have discussed, the hands have an extreme nervous sensitivity that carries the astral fluid, or double principle, to the brain where it gives birth to thought. Therefore, every impression we receive is implanted on the brain by the flow of the astral fluid. This flow can be rapid or slow. Because of this, every mental, emotional, and physical action, pleasant or unpleasant, affects our brain matter, at least for a time. Moreover, as the vital fluid flows from the fingertips to the brain and back again via the nervous system, the nervous system records these affects on our hands. This record remains long after the particular problem has dissipated.

It is the hands, then, that execute what the other senses can merely advise or prepare. When the astral fluid has entered the body, as we believe it does through the ends of the fingers, it becomes a prime motivator in establishing that the nose, eyes, and ears are able to perform their functions. It is at this moment that the hands receive their powerful gift and are able to do their part. When a child is born, it is apparent that hands are indispensable.

It is important to understand that a mudra is a living force that acts like a symbol. It is the realization and comprehension of a cosmic truth. Just as symbols are the language of the unseen, higher world, then, they are also the language of the subjective mind. Via the language of mudras or symbols, we can reach both the higher world and our own subjective mind.

Mudras are symbols that can directly affect the subconscious mind, arousing it into activity. In other words, symbols can be used to awaken realizations that lie dormant within the subjective mind. Again, some of these realizations have been dormant for several incarnations.

Spiritually-minded individuals, particularly Kabbalists, have always used symbols to decipher the mysteries of the material and immaterial worlds. Indeed, some mudras are tremendously powerful, as they are the charged language of the invisible world. The role of symbols is two-fold. The subconscious mind expresses itself with symbols and, conversely, symbols can be used to stimulate our subconscious mind. Symbols or mudras are the working tools of mystics. They are the thought forms of universal law. It is important to remember that mystical symbols or mudras are reflections in our consciousness of our discoveries in the astral realm. Life works both with symbols and manifests its continuous processes by way of symbols.

*The true purpose of life is to open your heart,
purging it of negative influences so that
you become a pure channel of God.*

*You are not here to glorify your little self,
for a candle that burns alone serves
only itself and its light slowly diminishes.*

*The burning candle that lights the path for others,
serves and uplifts the whole of humanity.
Its light becomes brighter and brighter.
Therefore, the true idea of life is to serve and
uplift others from the power of your Heart.*

2

NAAM YOGA AND UNIVERSAL KABBALAH

We attain success in our lives when we fit into the proper place. Therefore, we can attract success by attracting that open place that is right for us. In order to cause the opportunities that suit us perfectly to arise, we must first work on ourselves using the tools of Naam yoga and applying the laws of nature outlined in Universal Kabbalah. Then we must make ourselves universal in our thinking by realizing that we are one of God's multitude. The moment you attune yourself with this universal attitude, and stop viewing your life condition as something personal, is the moment you will begin to attract the success that is to be yours in this life. From the moment this realization takes hold, the floodgates of divine inspiration open to you. Your mind becomes clear, and your heart begins to listen. New messages come to you while you are chanting prayer, and you find that you are being led away from conditions that should not exist in your life. In this way you begin to experience favorable changes.

The knowledge of Universal Kabbalah and Naam yoga is everyone's birthright. The spiritual alchemy of combining these sacred and powerful traditions provides a seamless experience of life that permits the individual to master his/her destiny. Taken on its own, each discipline is rendered less powerful. For example, practicing the 84 yoga postures will lengthen your physical life, but they will not open your heart and bind you with God. It is through the practice of the Word that man merges with God, because God is bound by the Word. Naam yoga leads to cosmic consciousness primarily through the Naam. Naam yogis recite the Naam everyday until it becomes part of them, and they become part of it. By vibrating the Naam, they stimulate the base of the brain, so that consciousness can be achieved. The practice of the Word leads to the process of regeneration, which is the spiritual birth that results from the marriage of the conscious, the emotional and the intellectual. Universal Kabbalah accesses the power of the Word in the service of healing humankind. Working with the Word will give you an aura of irresistible attraction. The Word rebuilds both body and mind, making them purer and lighter than air. The Word gives you longevity, control of the thoughts and emotions, and balanced actions. It soothes the nervous system to the point where there is hardly any nervous tension left at all. This lends you a softness that is pleasantly magnetic to others. Old age recedes as the practice of the Word transforms the body into a vessel of purity with light shining from the face and eyes. Indeed, when you practice with the Word you retain a youthful, pleasant, attractive appearance. The Word rebuilds the mind, changing your concept of self and forcing your personality upward toward the Divine. It makes you think clearly and meditate better as it cultivates the desire to do good deeds.

When, by working with the Word, you realize that all humans are interconnected, your heart opens, and you become truthful and loving. You then strive to help others overcome their negativity. The Word lends great support to your circumvent force, thereby protecting you from negative and dark forces. As you learn to create and control this force, you are even able to change the destiny of others, for you can project this force to another's that may be weak, making their circumvent force strong enough to intercept the negative actions of the dark forces. In so doing, they are relieved of misfortune.

The importance of working with the Word cannot be overstated. It is vitally important, far more important than we realize. Chanting prayer is the bread of the soul. Prayer uplifts the soul. It is always necessary to pray. Praying is the art of using the Word with the intention of merging with God. When you pray, focus all your attention so that you awaken your spirit and the divine spark within you. Pray and ask for strength and the courage to overcome challenges. Pray before you sleep and when you first awaken, directing your soul toward God in each moment. Pray for those who don't understand their spirituality, for those who don't know how to connect with their spirit, and for those who cannot or will not do it, for your prayers can always assist those in darkness. If you find it is difficult to address God, the Father, invoke and implore the Queen of the heavens, Mary, and put yourself in her heart. As the human representative of the divine feminine principle, she will always intercede for you for the sake of her son.

When a musical instrument is out of tune, it creates discord. Similarly, when human beings are out of harmony with the divine order of things, we draw disharmony and disunity to us. Swimming against the tide, we exhaust ourselves but get nowhere. To keep yourself in tune and find your own note within the rhythm of life, you have to learn the art of vibrating the Word. The more you vibrate the Word, the more clearly you can reflect on the qualities of your soul. In turn, you will find that you are in harmony with yourself, and that internal harmony will be projected into your life. Once you are in tune with life, life flows smoothly. You do everything at the right time and everything falls perfectly into place. All you have to do is vibrate the Word so as to find your direct contact with the Creator. Then keep sounding your particular note loud and clear, and take your place within the vast orchestra of life. Miracle upon miracle will come about, and this way of living will become normal because you are in tune with God through the power of the Word.

As you rediscover your unique note within the vast orchestra of life as a result of working with the Word, God works in and through you to bring about His wonders and glories. It takes all kinds. Just as there are many different instruments in an orchestra, each of us has a rightful place within the whole. God breathes through everyone, good and bad. Therefore, do not judge and criticize others. Rather, focus on yourself and make sure that you play your own note. Do not seek to play another's, for those who seek to play someone else's note find themselves in disharmony with the whole. Indeed, when we go off on our own tangents with no thought or consideration for the whole, discord and chaos are created. Never try to be like anyone else or do what someone else is doing. Instead, take the time to readjust your energy, and be yourself. In so doing, your note will blend in perfectly with the harmony of the whole and life will become simple. Playing your right note can even help others. The tendency of the body of a lower rate of vibration is to strive to reach the higher rate of vibration. It is only a matter of time no matter how slow the progress may seem. Play your own note and there will no longer be any room for competition as you relax into being yourself. Learn to stand on your own two feet. Find your individual path and function in the overall plan.

We who practice both Naam yoga and Universal Kabbalah recognize that no one stream of truth leads to a comprehensive understanding of who and what the Divine truly is. Ours is a spiritual practice, not a religious one. In our modern, secular society, spirituality and religion are often viewed as synonymous. Spirituality, however, does not have a close relationship with any one religion. In fact, religious fanaticism is antithetical to spirituality. Spirituality is about values. Spirituality grants the self-knowledge that engenders tolerance, understanding, forgiveness, and eradicates selfishness. Those who take the time to offer help and consolation to one who has fallen by the wayside are living the spiritual life. Spirituality helps us to correct the errors we have committed and polishes the rough edges of our personality. We let go of the arrogance that knows too much, yet not enough; the pride that holds us above others and separates us from God; the cynicism that sees what is wrong with others and the world at large as it releases us from personal responsibility. Only by weaving together different strands of the existing traditions of divinity can humankind begin to conceive the true nature of the Divine. It is essential that more of the hidden truths of our various religious traditions and mystery systems be revealed, for this is the way humankind can begin to understand and relate to their source. In turn, we will gain a greater understanding of ourselves. Indeed, the time has come for the Divine Spiritual Wisdom to be shared in the spirit and service of helping humankind. As Universal Kabbalists, we understand that we do not weaken our power by passing on the truth. To the contrary, we are strengthened, for the generous are blessed and sanctified through their acts. In passing on the truth, we operate according to the principle that no human being has the right to judge the worthiness of others. That right is reserved solely for the Divine.

UNIVERSAL KABBALAH

What exactly is Universal Kabbalah? Universal Kabbalah is the sacred science through which the unknown becomes known, the unseen becomes seen, and the unheard becomes heard. It is an expression of the Divine's existence, and a map that allows us to see the face of God fragmented so as not to be blinded by the greater light. To be sure, Universal Kabbalah is a most valid and valuable map, worthy of much contemplation, for it is not only an external map that enables us to recognize the surreal consciousness of the Divine in our external world, it is also a mirror that enables us to see the Divine within ourselves. When we are able to see the various external and internal expressions of the Divine, we begin to recognize the states of consciousness that exist to help us draw ever closer to a personal discovery of divinity. We are then able to create healthy, effective lives. It must be said that the majority of men and women who study Universal Kabbalah have chosen the path of becoming both yogis and Kabbalists. Through the application of both spiritual disciplines, they have come to realize that there is a natural kinship between them. Moreover, they have attuned themselves to the unseen powers and forces of nature, as well as the universal laws that flow in, around, and throughout all of life. The spiritual technology of Universal Kabbalah has shown them how to work in accordance with these laws in order to achieve great success and contentment in their worldly experiences. Together, these men and women have formed an invisible empire of Naam yogis and Kabbalists that is expanding in America and other parts of the world.

Humankind desperately needs the Divine Spiritual Wisdom contained in Universal Kabbalah, for it is the tonic that soothes and heals all human infirmities. Ignorance is the worst and most potent form of disease, able to spawn a whole host of mental, emotional, and physical difficulties. That which removes the blinds of ignorance is the most potent of all medicines. Spiritual understanding destroys ignorance, for it leads to the revelation of the truth. It is the true healing power, the perfect medicine for individuals, groups, nations, and the globe. As the path based on entering into a state of unification with the Divine, Universal Kabbalah provides us with the spiritual understanding that removes the blinds of ignorance. Universal Kabbalah provides the practical tools and philosophical foundation that allows students to recognize the connection between the macrocosmic consciousness of the Source and the microcosmic consciousness of humankind. In recognizing this connection, our material and physical values are altered in a positive way as our capacity for wisdom increases exponentially. Remember, the unknown is merely that which has yet to be included within the consciousness of the seeker. When we are liberated from the bonds of ignorance, we are bathed in the radiance of light and understanding as to the purpose of existence. As the wisdom and goodness that permeates the whole of creation is made evident to our imperfect intellect, life, with all its joys and sorrows, becomes beautiful. We come to understand and master the three worlds, thereby increasing our capacity to know how to gradually incorporate the various elements of the universe within our being. Just think of the familial, social, and global changes that could occur, were we to all partake of the Divine Spiritual Wisdom! And were all to lead to the world of sacred wisdom, that land of peace where the finer qualities tucked away in the human soul are given the opportunity for expression, the breadth and calmness of truth would prevail.

The Divine Spiritual Wisdom that is Universal Kabbalah assists us in developing appreciation, as it reveals the glory of its knowledge and makes manifest the latent faculties that allow us to master the secrets of the seven spheres. For the Universal Kabbalist, the gates to the Mysteries lie within the heart. Central to Universal Kabbalah, then, is teaching us how to access our hearts and spiritualize our emotions. This is the key that unlocks the door of self-understanding and self-mastery. Knowledge of self is the secret to all knowledge we acquire, whether worldly or spiritual. Knowledge of self transforms, for once we have gained self-knowledge, we are able to make the changes necessary to refine our thoughts, motives, and behaviors. This movement from awareness to action is essential. Knowledge is useless unless one has the courage to put it into action. Once our emotions have been spiritualized, we are able to contact the more elevated plane, which is an essence that lives and breathes, both internally and externally, in all space and substance. Every man and woman houses two spheres, the lower non-self and the higher Self. These two spheres, that of the non-self with its concerns and that of the Self with its realizations, are connected by a gate. In the Universal Kabbalist, reason is the gate between the outer and the inner worlds. The mind illuminated by reason bridges the chasm between the corporeal and the incorporeal, thereby transforming the individual's concerns from those of men to those of gods.

As the student of Universal Kabbalah continues to delve more deeply into the spiritual principles governing the discipline, he/she gains insight into the workings of the universe and begins to embrace the Cosmic whole. Spirituality is enhanced to the point that it permeates the student's entire being in a concrete way that is beneficial to the student themselves, as well as everyone with whom he/she comes into contact. Moreover, the practice of Universal Kabbalah strengthens the individual's concept of faith. Faith is essential, for without faith life appears hopeless and our world appears devoid of fairness and goodness. Everything in life originates in Faith. Whatever you have Faith in will come to pass. If, for example, you have Faith in Love, you will experience Love. If you have Faith in strength, you will become strong. If you have Faith in Light and health, you will become healthy. But, Faith does not work in a vacuum. Faith needs Hope and Love. Hope, Faith, and Love are the most beautiful blanket of Light you can surround yourself with. They will break through any obstacle. All three are necessary, for Hope is the beginning of Faith. Faith is Hope and wisdom in action. Indeed, Faith is the Divine Spiritual Wisdom in action. The Divine Spiritual Wisdom is the combination of intelligence and truth on one pillar with Divine Love on the other pillar. Love is the living, visible manifestation of Hope and Faith. And, as with Hope and Faith, Love is essential, for goodness is the child of Love. Knowing and living Love will make you good. Hope is the catalyst. Without it you cannot have Faith and Love. Without Hope, then, you have nothing. Hope is intimately connected with the physical world. With regards to health, your level of health is dependent on your level of Hope. As you cannot consistently maintain strength without Faith, Faith also contributes directly to your level of health. The two pillars of which we speak are exceedingly important because to heal confusion you need the intelligence of the truth aspect of Divine Spiritual Wisdom. To heal fear and anger, you need the Divine Love aspect of the Divine Spiritual Wisdom. Above all, always remember that Hope, Faith, and Love in combination are the golden elixir that can remove all obstacles from your life.

Every time you are faced with a problem, keep in mind that the realization of the presence of God is the secret to removing it. It is the realization of the presence of God in the problem that you have which allows you to transmute whatever darkness you are facing into light. It is essential that we connect with the idea of a universal spiritual consciousness, with a God who makes all things possible. Otherwise, we cast ourselves into a world fraught with confusion, pain, and limitation. In such a world, ambitions are thwarted by the individual's inability to sustain inspiration, and success is only achieved through force or chance. Existing in the vacuum of egotism, the individual is unable to perceive anything beyond him/herself. This, of course, perpetuates the chaos of the world. The Universal Kabbalist is not troubled by the advantages and/or riches others may enjoy, for he/she understands that according to universal law, more must be given in order for more to be received. Indeed, according to the law of divine justice, we all receive exactly what we deserve. It is a gift from God and nature to mankind that those who deserve it may be compensated. He unto whom abundant wealth is given is selected to be the medium of distribution, or the distributor of nature's compensation. Regardless of the cause of one's fortunate position in life, whether through the influence of planetary bodies, whether obtained by the sweat of his brow or through a sudden acquisition of wealth, it is a fact that wealth received in excess of one's necessities is given for a definite purpose and must be used accordingly. If man is blessed at birth, or suddenly or slowly thereafter, with wealth, then nature expects that he will recompense life by using the blessings he has received to create the possibility of wealth for others. If he fails to carry out this mission, nature will deny him the joy he could have received from that wealth.

Nothing is done by chance. Our souls are sparks of the divine and examples of the creative principle itself. How then, can we believe that we are the product of chance? To do so engenders complacency and destroys all desire for progress and achievement. Our present environment may not be entirely to our liking, but we must always remember that life is a matter of perspective. In other words, a limited environment is not always a misfortune and an easy environment is not always a blessing. There is nothing in heaven or in existence that is not of God in some mysterious way. We must recognize God's presence in the darkest of nights as well as the brightest of days. We must recognize God's presence in the limited environment as well as the easy environment. We must recognize God's beauty in tragedy, adversity, or good fortune. Open your eyes to the wonder and presence of God, and alleviate the suffering of your stay here on earth. A limited environment, when viewed through the appropriate lens, provides incentive and stimulates ambition. Moreover, by not lending itself to distraction, a limited environment can prevent the individual from getting off course. On the other hand, an environment of ease and wealth requires that the individual access great stability of character and firmness of purpose in order to make the most of themselves and rise to great heights.

Accept your present life circumstances just as they are. Do not worry about the past causes that precipitated your lot in this life. Instead, concentrate on today by living in the here and now. In this way, you will be better able to regard your life as simply the raw material with which you have to work with. No matter how humble or restricted, you can make your life a thing of joy and beauty.

Living a spiritual life means loving God above all, and your neighbor as yourself. As a Universal Kabbalist, it is incumbent upon you to follow this mandate, regardless of your lot in life. Loving God and your neighbors is the motive of will, and the essence of Love is the Christic light in us. The principle of new life exists in this twofold love. Good lies in the love you have for God and your neighbor, and through serving others. You must know no love other than the love of all, know no interest other than the interest of all, and know no well being other than the well being of all. As God gives, so too must we give. When you give you become God, and Good. The holy scriptures ask us to regard all beings with neutrality and to help each living thing, no matter their stature or sin. Practice true charity, and the heavens will listen to you. The

Universal Kabbalist knows that the seed of good lies within all, no matter how evil someone may appear at first glance. Armed with such knowledge, he/she has faith that in the course of spiritual development the seed of good will grow and blossom.

As the Universal Kabbalist always seeks the light of truth, he/she prefers the company of those who know its value. By working with the Sun and associating with good spiritual people, he/she finds his/her way out of the darkness of ignorance. He/she is aware that mixing with those who only love social gatherings is a waste of time and energy, while mixing with those who love God will enhance his/her love of God. As he/she strives for growth in all dimensions of his/her being, the Universal Kabbalist remains naturally humble. He/she does not need or want to demonstrate the possession of spiritual gifts that have been acquired. Rather, he/she keeps the majority of his/her wisdom locked in his/her heart, knowing that true power lies in silence. The greater the Universal Kabbalist's gifts, the greater is his/her modesty and will to obey the laws of nature. For he/she who truly becomes one with God has no need to prove to himself/herself or others the extent of the power he/she possesses. He/she knows within that he/she has all powers at his/her command, and that there is nothing to fear. The Universal Kabbalist, then, uses his/her power only when God has directed him/her to do so.

Our work is pure theurgy and is considered the supreme work. Its source has been received from the higher worlds of the unseen, thereby creating a hierarchy that extends from the higher world down to our lower world. This supreme work can only manifest through the agency and simplicity of prayer, along with the sacrifice that comes from service. People tend to think that God is in the head, when in fact God is hidden in the heart of the humble and simplest man. Universal Kabbalists pray and apply the precepts of the Christic light in their daily lives, for this keeps the darkness that blinds and disrupts at bay. As long as we are in darkness, we cannot see or feel anything, but the moment we live in light, we can see and feel everything. Therefore, we pray to light the candle of our heart and get rid of darkness so that everything may work.

The moment a person is enlightened, he/she may not be understandable to others. The reason is fear of change. When one becomes enlightened, both the atmosphere and approach change. Universal Kabbalah assists us by providing the practical tools and life philosophy of service to others that reminds us that we are, in essence, spiritual beings having a human experience. There is no greater power than that which arises from the constructive and compassionate use of knowledge, and no greater confidence than that which is born of understanding. Again, central to the belief system of Universal Kabbalists is developing the ability to think universally. As we have stated, this is a crucial concept, for equality is all God and Nature understand. Universal Kabbalists recognize that we are all God's children. God never segregated us according to race, ethnicity, or nationality. These categories are the effects of climate, evolution, and conditions that have been descending on human beings since the dawn of creation. Nor did God create religion; it is a man-made construct that has been thrust upon us. Furthermore, God did not make delineations about which people should automatically be considered good and worthy, and those who should be considered bad and unworthy. All prejudicial claims—women are inferior to men, one race is superior to another, one way of living is better than all others, have no place in the mind of the Universal Kabbalist, for he/she understands that Divine essence runs, like a stream, through all mortals. The true Universal Kabbalist, then, is neither narrow-minded nor restrictive in either word or deed; he/she treats everyone kindly and is always ready to offer a helping hand. He/she is universal, like the Sun, that power that governs and gives life to the whole of the universe. By maintaining universality he/she continually reestablishes the link between the Sun and him/herself. As a result, all the separate pieces of his/her life come together in the rhythm of universal life, and he/she experiences the grace of God.

Universal consciousness is the way of light, the way of the Sun, and the way of the heart. Those who do not think universally spend their lives competing in the hard-hearted game of winner take all. This leads to a life of misery and emptiness where duality reigns supreme. An inability to think universally leads to the creation of superiority complexes that, in turn, create the possibility for you to experience misfortune. Presently, the Earth is vibrating at the frequency of group consciousness, making those who vibrate in individual consciousness miserable. Group consciousness comes through service, and will make you comfortable in this age. But what does it truly mean to think and live universally? Those who are universal live in universal consciousness. They have moved from individual consciousness to group consciousness, and then to universal consciousness. They know that all is light. In other words, these individuals are evolved enough to recognize the light in everyone and everything, for everyone and everything is a crystallization of the light of the Sun. Wise are those who keep in mind that we all originate from the One that created all, and will return to the One that created all. The One that created all lives in each of us. As soon as a person feels that he/she is part of Infinity, and that Infinity is part of him/her, his/her limitations will cease and grace and happiness will flow. The secret of happiness and good health is to be One with the One. We are One, from the One. Our purpose is to be One with the One. One knows we are One, and all the creation is One. We are One with all creation. All creation is with the One. One created One, and One is within One, and within all aspects of One remains One. In the beginning was the One. Now is the One. In the end will be One. Learn to see God in yourself, in others, and in all teachings, for this leads to a real understanding of how interconnected we all are. As Universal Kabbalah maintains, if you cannot see God in all, you cannot see God at all.

The key to our collective salvation and reintegration is in the recognition that we are all children of the same Father, God, and the same Mother, Nature, or the Universal Soul. Until we realize this, we will never understand our true nature. Collectively, man will continue to be out of touch with the essential core of reality, suffering in the self-imposed slavery of ignorance. The fastest way out of the mire of our own ignorance is the Divine Spiritual Wisdom, for it teaches us the means of helping, uplifting, and serving others who may still be trapped by their own blindness, as it simultaneously ensures that we heal and enhance ourselves and our work. It is imperative that we realize that our individual and collective mission is to bring the talents and virtues of Heaven, sown within our souls, to full bloom. We must constantly strive for perfection of the self. After a series of individual liberations have occurred, the great collective liberation can take place. This will allow for the reconstitution of the Archetype and its reintegration into the Divine. Once abandoned by its animator, and left to the anarchic nature of fallen spirits, the material world will dissolve at an accelerated pace thus signaling the end of the physical universe as foretold by all the great traditions.

Presently, man may live two lives. The first is measured by our own creation, time, and is the struggle from the womb to the tomb. It can be called the unheeding life. The second is from realization to infinity. This life, consummated on the plane of eternity, begins with understanding, and its duration is forever. This is the way of life adhered to by Universal Kabbalists and it requires that one maintain good health on all levels. The Universal Kabbalist understands that the basic ingredients of good health are mental, and not physical. In most cases where the inharmonious symptoms of illness manifest in the physical body, the fundamental cause is the expression of a destructive emotion such as jealousy, hatred, envy, injustice, suspicion, anger, and greed, all of which, of course, originate in the mind. Birthed by self-centeredness, they are barriers to spiritual growth and prevent man's escape from the misery of soul ignorance. When faced with challenging mental, emotional, or physical states of being, the Universal Kabbalist remains steady in his/her attunement with the universe and adherence to living in harmony with natural and spiritual laws. In this way, he/she can invoke heavenly help in whatever he/she wishes to accomplish. Furthermore, in living in such a manner, the Universal Kabbalist is recognizable for the positive and uplifting vibrations he/she radiates, for he/she has developed the strength and courage necessary to manifest only that which is in tune with the infinite. The Universal Kabbalist is alive with the purifying, vitalizing, healing forces of the universe to such an extent that his/her life becomes an expression of strength, serenity, prosperity, and health. In turn, his/her vision becomes clearer, his/her heart happier, and his/her person richer in numerous ways. In short, the Universal Kabbalist strives to maintain good health, and is aware that the key to good health lies in obedience to the laws of nature. The word law connotes power and control. It is the rule of law that makes the universe so entirely dependable. This dependability, evident in the Sun's daily rise above the horizon, allows human beings to plan a calendar a century in advance, predict eclipses of the Sun and Moon with accuracy, and chart a schedule of the ocean's tides. Indeed, natural and universal law allow for the very life and growth of the planet and its inhabitants. If we accept that natural and universal law is the cornerstone of the universe, it follows that law governs every phase of human development. When we study natural and universal law, we gain knowledge, power, and wisdom. Knowing and understanding the laws of life releases us from fear. Within these laws lie the tools that aid us in creating something beautiful with our lives, just as the musician uses his instrument to create music. All we need to do is utilize all the principles our sages have discovered and tested, for by the knowledge of the laws of nature, we honor nature.

It must be said that a truly spiritual being disciplines him/herself to become successful in the material world while concurrently moving toward spiritual attainment. While maintaining this balance requires effort, it is critical. One cannot allow him/herself to become materialistic to the point where spirituality is neglected. The spiritual person does not let business pursuits cause him/her to violate his/her moral precepts or the dictates of his/her conscience. Moreover, he/she does not let material interests deprive him/her of opportunities for introspection, reflection, and study. Remember, one's degree of spirituality is based upon the things he/she values. Material objects are transitory. Life's real value is found in living purposefully, and in developing the spirituality of our being. Having said that, one cannot live in the world of abstract ideas to the point of not meeting his/her material needs. The spiritual person needs not sacrifice his/her common sense; it will serve him/her well. Man is not measured by the quantity of his acts, but by their quality. The individual who subscribes to and lives by spiritual ideals and principles is directing his/her life in useful channels and constructive activities. He/she has a full realization of Divine nature, and the way he/she thinks, feels, speaks, and acts reveals his/her philosophy of life in its entirety. Simply put, to be spiritual means to live life with a spiritual technology that permeates all thoughts, words, and deeds. One of the greatest weaknesses of humankind is our dependence upon our fellow man for assistance in surmounting the unfortunate conditions that we, ourselves, have precipitated. It is when we learn to take responsibility for ourselves by subordinating our passions and transforming our animalistic nature that the spiritual principles that lie dormant within will rise up and become dominant in our consciousness, thereby leading to peace in the world. Take care, then, to respect and enhance both the physical and spiritual sides of your nature. Otherwise, you will become imbalanced and enslaved by your own pronouncements.

As Universal Kabbalists, it is our sacred duty collectively and individually to lead humankind forward, past the swamps of religion, creed, race, color, class, and gender into the new age where, through a realization of our common original estate, we may find the strength to reconcile our differences, and the courage to dwell in harmony. The extent to which we learn the Divine Spiritual Wisdom and develop ourselves, is the extent to which we will help lift the race. To develop yourself is to raise your frequency. To raise your frequency is to influence everyone with whom you come into contact, for it is only a matter of time before the positive thoughts within you permeate your community. We must set the example and create the milieu. We must influence the cultural atmosphere of our circle. Raise your standards, and open your heart, mind, and soul to all that is true, good, and harmonious. Become an oasis of inspiration and hope for those who seek your counsel. Never reject someone in need, for the breath of God emanates from every human being. Be compassionate, because each virtuous act is rewarded one hundredfold. Be philanthropic; if you have a surplus, share it with others because God asks us to share the fortune we have been given by Him with those who are bereft. Don't worry about your next meal; focus instead on whether your neighbor ate today. Do not waste your resources; God has provided amply for your material life. Do not be guilty of throwing out the bread on your table to acquire fresh bread. Remember that another living being who is starving may still be nourished by it. Give spontaneously and generously from your heart without expectations. Realize that the beggar who has misused what has been given to him is responsible for the karma he creates. Do good deeds, but do so anonymously so as to relinquish all ego attachment. Your right hand must not know what your left hand is doing.

God never forgets His children. Each of us has been given a guardian angel who follows us from the womb to the tomb. When we are vain or believe we are in complete control of our lives, we pollute our connection with the angel we have been granted. In so doing, we potentially hamper our ability to receive heavenly intervention. When, however, we are humble and pray we provide our guardian angel with the opportunity to guide us and awaken our highest instincts. All God asks is that we apply every effort to becoming a good person. Strive to be a good person and to correct your mistakes, for heaven will only forgive you after your debts have been paid. Learn to give of yourself and sacrifice for the higher good. Face violence with compassion, evil with good, and judgment with love, and you will inspire people to choose the right path. Always try to transform evil into good. Remember, evil exists to give us the means to become good soldiers of Heaven so that we may acquire strength for future fights. Pray for your enemies because they are miserable. They do not know what they are doing, and you do not know what harm you may have caused in previous lives. Along your path you will never meet those who have the power to remove your sins if you have caused a tremendous amount of damage to others. Forgive the trespasses of others so that you may enter the Kingdom of Heaven. Do not seek vengeance. Rather, forgive the evil that has been done to you and you will plant the seeds of goodness in your enemies. Ignore gossip and negative criticism, because those who sully your reputation only make it brighter by purifying you under the heavens. Love with the highest, unconditional intention, and not with an expectation of being loved in return. Love without ownership and cherish without attachment.

Everything in life is simple. May each moment of your life be an act of faith, of gracious simplicity in action. Follow the Christic path and you will always live in the truth, for Christic Master has shown us the way to the heart of God. The Christic Master has walked the path to heaven, a path full of challenges, to open the door to heaven for us all. When we rise above the incessant voice of the ego, we remember at each moment that we are nothing but the instrument of a heaven to which we are grateful for all our gifts and graces. Respect the celestial hierarchy, which manifests here on earth through the spiritual community to which you belong. Make it your aim to abide by the laws of your respective country while obeying the natural laws of the universe. Assist those in distress with tact, silence, and discretion. Attempt to do good work without bringing attention to yourself. Seek truth, open your consciousness to follow the Christic path, and merge with Divine Spiritual Wisdom so as to radically alter your life.

The Ancients have left us a heritage of Divine Spiritual Wisdom by which peace may be attained. Each of us must strive, however, to live in accordance with the teachings of our sacred wisdom. Heal yourself by working with the laws of nature. In so doing, you will affirm your divinity and create the conditions for spiritual and material success. This is a truth understood by Universal Kabbalists. Humanity has striven after truth for ages, and yet there has never been a period in the history of the world in which some men have not realized the truth. The mystic's view is, what I have known today has been known before, and will be known afterwards. It has never been known by all, and will never be known by all. But, as the sight becomes keen, so man will be able to see. Universal Kabbalah provides all the tools you will need to gain self-mastery, which is of great assistance as we attempt to surmount and mitigate the problems we find in our environment and circumstances. This is the essence of life-mastery. Together, self-mastery and life-mastery create balance in every area of our lives. By the knowledge of self, may we master self, and by the improvement of self may we improve mankind. As you begin the journey that is Universal Kabbalah, keep in mind that the spiritual path does not always bring a life of ease, for physical life was not intended to be a joy ride, but rather a vehicle whereby we could reconcile our karma and make our way back to our True Home. The spiritual path will, however, bring the strength of character we need to overcome life's obstacles with objectivity, faith, and hope. It adjusts our thoughts, words, and deeds so that we can attract what we need and move gracefully through the challenges of this time in human history.

Universal Kabbalah helps us, as it provides the practical means whereby we can improve our personality and develop our talents. By employing this sacred science, you are able to develop your mind and summon the courage to rise above your environment. As you develop neutrality, you are able to ignore those who seek to undermine your confidence and faith. You will begin to smile at criticism and disapproval. At the same time, your circle of friends and acquaintances will enlarge. All true Universal Kabbalists attract others through their optimistic outlook on life, their zest for living, their courageousness in rising above the difficulties and restrictions of their environment, their insatiable curiosity for experience and knowledge, their intense interest in the problems of their community and the world, and their love of life, man, and God. Others come to us and discover for themselves the faith that sustains us and keeps us young. Not only are we magnetic to others, we come to attract the beneficent forces of the universe. In us the blessings of the scriptures are fulfilled. We shall be as the children of Heaven, loving and pursuing peace, and acting as a blessing to all who know us.

Universal Kabbalists understand that obeying the laws of life and applying spiritual understanding brings health, contentment and peace of mind. They understand that by harmonizing their thinking with the spiritual laws of our sacred wisdom, they are on their way toward lives of love, peace, light, and health. Moreover, they understand that, as true Kabbalists and yogis, they are neither born nor do they die, for they have achieved the realization of immortality through communion with the Self. Having come to the realization that there exists an immortal foundation that will not pass away, they themselves have become immortal. They erect a civilization, on the vibrant base that is the Self, which will endure after the sun, moon, and stars have been extinguished. The universe has provided a space, an opening, for each of us to live and flourish on all planes of existence. Employ the tools of Universal Kabbalah and claim yours. Remember, the fool lives only for today, the true Kabbalist and/or yogi lives forever.

Meditation for Attracting the Energy of Jupiter

POSITION:
Sit straight in easy pose. Eyes are opened 1/10 and focused at the tip of the nose.

Hold your hands in *Sarab Gyan Mudra*, in front of the heart center. The fingers are interlocked with the index fingers pointing up and thumbs crossed. The arms are relaxed.

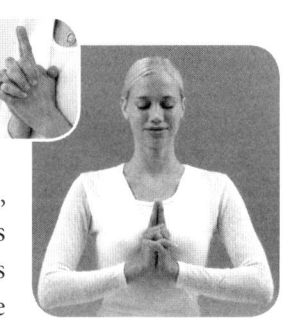

MANTRA:
Har Haray Haree
Wahe Guru (pronounced *Wha-hey Guroo*)

(Optional: Chant along with Track #2 of the Green House CD)

TIME: Continue for 11 minutes. To end, inhale deeply, suspend the breath and relax.

COMMENTS:
This mudra brings a sense of self-containment because the hands are interlocked at the heart center. It evokes the expansion from the planet Jupiter, the index finger. Jupiter stands for the sphere Chesed on the Tree of Life. It is the flow of divine grace through which the creation is effected. In Hebrew Chesed means *mercy*. This is the house of Dharma. Jupiter, who is the lord of wellness, stands for abundance, authority and generosity. Jupiter bestows material and spiritual wealth. Practice this posture with this most exalted mantra and these qualities of God will manifest in your psyche.

Meditation for Maturity and Wisdom

Position:
Sit in easy pose with the spine straight. Gently focus the eyes at the tip of the nose.

With the elbows down by your sides, extend the forearms up so that the palms are a few inches in front of each shoulder, palms flat and facing the body. Then slightly bend the wrists, until the palms are facing up and are somewhat relaxed and cupped. Just hold this position.

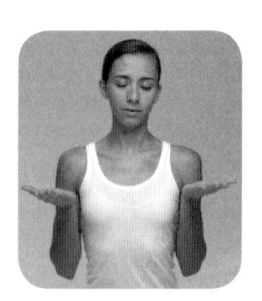

Movement:
Without using the breath in any specific way, begin to pump the navel point powerfully. Pump very hard and fast. (This is not Breath of Fire.)

Time:
Continue for 31 minutes. To end, inhale and pump the navel vigorously. Hold 10 seconds. Exhale. Repeat 3 times total. Relax.

Comments:
This meditation builds the circumvent force and the ability to attract goodness, while awakening your life true potential. The more powerful one is, the more one should serve others. Make yourself so powerful and increase the light of God in you, so that things may not bother you, and your peace may not be shaken. So, it is very beautiful for one to drop the past, change attitude, have an altitude, and make sense to oneself. Then, everybody can understand that you are beautiful, bountiful, and blissful, trustworthy, gracious, with divinity and dignity, and you can be a friend unto Infinity. You must understand: there is no prize that can give you back your honor.

Harmonize the Brain for Maximum Effectiveness

POSITION:
Sit in easy pose with the spine straight. Eyes are closed. Bring the hands up in front of the shoulders and move them a little out to the sides. Palms are flat with the fingers pointing straight up towards the ceiling. Split the fingers between the middle and ring fingers, keeping the index and middle fingers pressed side-by-side. Extend the thumbs straight out away from the rest of the hand. Maintain the finger-split.

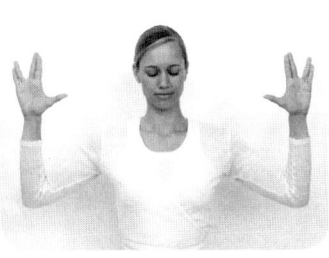

MANTRA:
Aad Such – Jugaad Such – Haibhee Such – Naanak Hosee Bhee Such

BREATH:
Inhale through the nose in 10 equal strokes. Hold the breath in and repeat the chant mentally. Then exhale through the nose in 10 equal deliberate strokes. Hold the breath out and repeat the chant mentally. Establish an inner attitude of grace and regality.

TIME: Continue for 11 to 31 minutes. Inhale deeply and relax.

COMMENTS: This meditation opens the stimulation of the brain. Both hemispheres communicate and integrate to initiate the meditative mind. It creates a window through which you can project the mind and travel in the many worlds of the creation. Normally the brain does not function at its highest capacity. Just as it takes special exercise to develop the musculature of the body, so too do we need special exercises to develop the mind. We usually live in a very narrow range of perception, like a perceptual jail. We need a systematic technique to chip away at that prison and to experience a greater world beyond our perceived world. This expansion of worlds is not mystical and mysterious; it only seems that way when there is no mastery and no experience of the inner reality and infinity of the self in God.

Understand that man has,
within himself, the manifested God.
We call it the soul.
The sole purpose of life is to
activate the dormant soul.
When a ray of light mixes with real light,
the whole world becomes light.
A drop merged with the ocean
becomes the oceans.

3

DIVINE SPIRITUAL WISDOM

This century will bear witness to an amazing epoch in history, for the majesty of this sacred science will illuminate and clarify certain spiritual mysteries in order to facilitate the evolution of our physical world. Indeed, we are approaching the time when the great gates that protect the holies of holies will be lifted. Now is the time in which greater truths concerning the nature of the Divine Spiritual Wisdom will be brought forward and explained in greater detail. We are approaching a time when the heart will unite with the head, and man will unite with God. We are approaching the realm of love, peace, and light. We are approaching the realm of wisdom and the realm of God, the source of light. Therefore, we invite you to join this holy group in which the Spirit of Wisdom itself will guide and teach all who approach it with a genuine thirst for knowledge. As you become a devotee of our sacred science, you will possess all the virtues, riches, and graces that God will bestow upon you, and celestial and terrestrial creatures will serve you in the accomplishment of the great work. This work will give you an experience of your own strength, your own purity, and your own infinity. Indeed, via our sacred wisdom, your life will become one of radiance. This sacred wisdom will cause the sun of light and truth to rise and pass over your life, banishing all shadows with the directness of its rays. The first ray of light breaks through the cloud of the mystery, announcing the coming of the Sun of wisdom and its treasure. Under the tutelage of these sacred teachings, Divinity bends to humankind so that it may externally write the Truth that is an interior and eternal mystery upon his soul. The Divine Spiritual Wisdom possesses the keys to all mysteries, and grants insight and understanding of the innermost part of nature and creation. Within it you'll find the meaning of all spiritual symbols and rituals as well as the inner truths of all sacred books. By lifting the veil that blankets your soul, our sacred teachings give you a clearer vision of your life's purpose. As you discover your reason for being here, direct all your endeavors to the honor of God. This is how you will learn to rule over all the earth, as well as work in tandem with celestial beings, such as angels, who you will invoke and kindly release according to your will, to create great works. You will learn how to heal yourself, uplift others, and help in a positive evolution of humankind. The Divine Spiritual Wisdom that flows from Universal Kabbalah improves your life, restores your health, solves the many problems of your existence, and leads to happiness. These abilities make it authentic. This heavenly science is a real science, founded on pure and genuine truth. It is the promised inheritance of the elect who are capable of light and the golden path for all who want to achieve self-healing, serve others, and contribute to the positive evolution of humankind. It is imperative for us to realize that our individual and collective mission is to bring all the talents and virtues of Heaven that have been sown in us into full bloom. We are meant to live the life of our spiritual soul, and must strive to do so. There is no joy equal to the joy of learning and working with the Divine Spiritual Wisdom. Once you have tasted the sweetness that is your birthright, you will want nothing else.

    Most people who wish to understand the invisible world dabble in magic to obtain personal power. Then, as they evolve, they cease their pursuit of magic, because they realize that it has little efficacy and only tells a fraction of a much greater and more beautiful story of life. Kabbalah is not a matter of head, it is a matter of heart. Your head makes you individual, and your heart makes you universal. But even beyond the head and the heart, it is you. Just know that you are not the soul, you are not the mind, you are not the body. You are the controller of the three. You are the driving force of the three, to cover the distance and the destiny. You have a nervous system, a glandular system, and a circulatory system, the rejuvenation of the cell system, a liver to rebuild and filter things, and you have a spleen. The whole machine is so complicated, but so simple. In the kingdom of God everything happens naturally and simply. In order to understand this simplicity one must have a pure and unclouded conception of God, nature, and man. Understand that the Divine Spiritual Wisdom is complete and whole. It is the spiritual art and science whose truth has been divided in order to create various religions. Any religion, then, is merely a branch on the tree of the Divine Spiritual Wisdom. These branches must once again merge, thereby moving from divisive multiplicity to the unity of one Great Sacred Science. In ancient times, the temples of the spirit were visible in the material world, but because a pervasive lack of spirituality now exists, these temples have been rendered invisible to our external sight. The most elevated truths are clothed in an impenetrable veil because we have not been ready to receive them. Yet and still, as long as the human race has walked the earth there has always been a safe method of connecting with the unseen world.

The time to see the God of Abraham, Moses, and King Solomon as the necessity of life is now. Man must merge with the Lord and rise beyond his deficiencies and the dark shackles of negative behaviors and mechanical routines in order to tap into the source of all power and fulfillment. Man can have no power to act, feel or think without God. The truth is that without the true opening of the heart, which brings inner satisfaction, no amount of external good fortune can bring lasting peace of mind and heart. Our Divine Spiritual Wisdom teaches us how to rise above the delusion of separation and realize our oneness with God, to regain the lost paradise of consciousness by which man knows that he is, and ever has been, one with spirit. Man has it within his power to perfect himself and, in time, to undergo complete transformation. However, this transfiguration must take place in the innermost self, in the deepest ways we think, feel, and act each moment of each day. Working with our spiritual wisdom will make you calm and relaxed, happy and peaceful. The sacred teachings will quench your thirst for knowledge and uplift your heart, putting a smile upon your face and laughter in your voice. Let God work through you, through your hand, your feet, and your will. Embrace these teachings deep in your heart. Develop a spiritual discipline based upon the mantric science, or the way of the Sun. Meditate on God and work on yourself. As your whole demeanor changes from the inside out, you will be a source of inspiration to others even as you are inspired by the life around you.

This sacred science will unveil to you secrets you have never even imagined. It will expand your perception and give you an experience of your own infinity so that you may experience your vastness and enjoy your life. It will give you the blissful experience of the energy from above. As you begin to traverse the bridge between the physical and the spiritual, you will learn to perceive the physical world with different eyes. You can then take your new energy and sacred wisdom and employ it in the service of helping others to widening their perception. During this time on the planet, it is especially important that we endeavor to devote time to these sacred teachings. This sacred system will cause you to know yourself, to believe in yourself, to understand your power and lean on your strength, and to connect with your divinity. These sacred teachings will help you move through life in a healthy manner, in greater wisdom, harmony and serenity with yourself and with everyone on the planet. No longer will you be the victim of circumstances in time and space; instead, you will gain the courage to take true responsibility for your life, and act with grace and dignity. Indeed, our sacred science bestows the spiritual nobility and mystic sublimity that makes us beloved by heart centered people and feared by the enemies of light and divine knowledge.

If you want to acquire knowledge of the divine spiritual sciences, you must absorb all the information available to you and work within the appropriate spiritual guidelines. This is how you arrive at the desired end. For example, it is propitious to invoke the spirits on the days and hours when they have power and absolute empire. Students who read Lifting the Veil and join the Self Study course will understand such concepts as the intrinsic properties of the planets and the angels who serve them, to what angel each day and hour is submitted, along with their corresponding colors, the complementary metals, herbs, plants, aquatic, aerial, terrestrial beings, as well as the quarter of the universe where they ask to be invoked. You must apply all that information so as to create the purest line of contact with these angels. It cannot be stressed enough that this sacred work is for those who seek the Truth with a good and honest heart. Rediscover your Divine Nature so that you may celebrate Love, Light, and Liberty with Us. Work with the wisdom of the Ages to affect positive planetary transformation.

Our sacred wisdom helps you understand the application and implication of its time proven truths and demonstrates the effectiveness of the Word. Unfortunately, the average man will not understand the depth and effectiveness of working with the Word. However, the use of the Word is a timeless, simple truth that allows you to gracefully face the challenges of time and space. This, the greatest power of man, is completely at your disposal. As you absorb this Divine Spiritual Wisdom, your consciousness expands and you are filled with so much light that you become unshakable. You receive a whole host of benefits, as well as the guidance and help you need to experience a happy, successful, and fulfilling life. Journey to this golden path and breathe the healing wisdom, so that you may bathe in the heart of God. Project the radiant beauty of your inner self. Let the gift of this sacred science help you remove any remaining spiritual obstacles and enable your dazzling cosmic energy to reach as far as possible in the universe. Let the Divine Spiritual Wisdom make the sun of your destiny bright and the sky of your life clear and blue. However, as you learn this sacred science and practice with the Word, always remember that the tools with which we have been blessed belong to our Creator. All things come from God, and all things go to God.

In the eyes of the material world, the Divine Spiritual Wisdom may be seen as folly because it demonstrates, through personal experience, that the world itself is a folly. Indeed, the seekers of truth who return to the self-healing path of wisdom are ignorantly perceived as fools by those who live in darkness. Understand that man has, within himself, the manifested God. We call it the soul. The sole purpose of life is to activate the dormant soul. When a ray of light mixes with Light, the whole world becomes Light. A drop merged with the ocean becomes the oceans. These chanting prayers in our sacred teachings are the seals and service is the key.

Those who refuse to serve others are abandoned by the heavens. When we lose our ego through our true charity, we truly become the children of heaven. Regardless of what your mission is on the earth, remember to be humble. When you are convinced of your own importance, you cannot accomplish anything at all, because the heavens only come to the rescue of the weak, the humble, and those who serve others. The meek are always supported by God. The purpose of this life on earth is to have peace of mind and heart. The Divine Spiritual Wisdom gives us peace of mind and heart through the Word; our true work is the science of adaptation through the way of the heart. The heart is located in the chest, the root of the electro-magnetic field and the center of feeling. Feelings are the only true creator on all planes. Ideas are only creative on the human mental plane and can only reach the superior nature of the heavens with difficulty based on their crudeness. Prayer is the great mystery, and allows one to receive the highest influence in action on the divine plane through the Word made flesh, or the Christic force.

We also believe that we can activate an esoteric baptism within ourselves that purifies us in the eyes of God. Its mark does not exist in this world; it is an indelible mark that the Christ himself places in our hearts. As a result, the Christic force speak through our voice, and uplift others through our presence. We believe in the baptism of the heart by the Word. We are ready to follow the way of the heart, for the heavens have prepared us for it.

Those who learn this sacred science and practice with the Word become blessed and overcome their past karmas. There are two types of Kabbalists: those who practice Kabbalah with the help of a magical material device such as a wand, string, or talisman, and those who practice Kabbalah using nothing but the power of the Word. Tradition tells us that in the past, man knew how to create through the power of the Word. In this distant past, external objects were not necessary. It was only when man committed the first sin, thereby separating himself from God and becoming increasingly more immersed in matter, that he lost this power and was obliged to use his hand to create. Speech remains, however, man's true sword. Any material instrument, no matter how magical, can be lost because it is external. The Word, on the other hand, is internal and spiritual and, therefore, can never be lost. The Caduceus belongs to Mercury, the god of magic, and Mercury rules words, the mouth and the hands.

Words are extremely powerful, but in order to use them to transform your being and environment, you must gain mastery of your speech, feelings, and thoughts. Indeed, control of the Word is one of the primary requirements of the spiritual life, for without devotion to God and love of the Word there can be no spiritual growth. The Word must be an uplifting, healing intellectual gift to those with whom we interact. In this way we may add to their light and virtue. The Word must focus on spiritual truths, for the Word is the light of infinity that should be ever increasing. By chanting prayer, refraining from all forms of negativity, and serving others, we can recapture the power of the Word. As the God within takes control of your Word, an inner alchemy occurs whereby passion is transmuted into compassion, lust into love, and antipathy into sympathy. When you learn and work with the Divine Spiritual Wisdom, you are learning the healing mathematics of spirituality. Such work brings balance in your head, which is reproduced in your entire being. Intellectual gymnastics and philosophical discourse will not create an ideal life. Practicing the Word is the only way to attain an ideal life, and the only hope for the regeneration and restoration of the human dignity we have lost. The Divine Spiritual Wisdom will save you from all mental, spiritual, physical, past, present, and future darkness. It takes care of all mental and physical sickness. Understand that the purpose of every moment of life in the material realm is to acquire the wisdom, strength, and virtue that comes from working with the sacred science. Anything that is not of the sacred wisdom only debases humankind. Armed with the Divine Spiritual Wisdom and the power of the Word, we become well-suited for the sentiments of nature, lawful pleasures, and all virtues. In the absence of these most potent of spiritual tools, our hearts remain petrified.

As we move from the Age of Pisces to the Age of Aquarius, and the Heavens are re-positioning themselves, we must keep in mind that, this is the age of experience and spirituality. Unfortunately, most people have not yet focused their energies on spiritual development and, therefore, only experience the material plane of existence. Only those with the Divine Spiritual Wisdom who are practicing with the Word, will be effective in their lives. It is these people who will be called to heal and uplift others. As a result they will be liked, respected, understood, and confided in. The Word is the greatest weapon we have as we strive to overcome the damage of the past. Knowing and vibrating the Word is a scientific way of relating to God through the balance, combination, and permutation of sound. Keep in mind that in the beginning there was only sound. That sound made a point of energy then split into two to assume a shape similar to the figure eight. This was consciousness plus energy, and it was the beginning of creation, a time of pure bliss. The universe took form when bliss was overpowered by creative energy. Eventually ignorance overpowered creative energy, and desires and attachment were born to sustain the world.

Always remember that in the beginning was the Word. Work with the Word. The power of the Saints of God goes to those who meditate on the Word. And, meditating on the Word bestows the blessing and seven gifts of the Holy Ghost. Those who know and revere the Word shall know God. The Word stimulates your entire spiritual body, making you divine. For those who have perfected the Word, there is no miracle that cannot be manifested. Indeed, you can manifest anything and everything when you perfect the Word. Recite the Word every day until it becomes part of you, and you become part of it. Always remember, you shall be protected as long as you learn the Divine Spiritual Wisdom and vibrate the Word. By vibrating the Word, we stimulate the base of the brain, so that Consciousness can be achieved. Mastery of the Word grants spiritual growth. The Divine Spiritual Wisdom is the path of man to God, and God to man. This is the path that allows you to know the unknown. It is important for us to realize that the unknown is the totality, while the known is confinement. Therefore, the known must find, know, and understand the unknown. In other words, the known must experience and deal with the unknown. This is how true happiness is achieved, for knowing the unknown will give you radiance, self-confidence, equilibrium, balance, and stability, as well as carry you through any adversity.

The guardian and healing angel of this age is Guru Ram Das. The healing power of *Ra Ma Da Sa Sa Say So Hung*, the basic healing energy and sound current of Ram Das, is in the *RaMaDaSa* CD. In order to increase and expand on the opportunities that come into your life, use the latest *Green House* CD. The *Soul Trance* CD eases anxiety and depression, and initiates emotional healing. Use *RaMaDaSa* to heal yourself and others. Work with the *Heaven's Touch* CD to synchronize your energy and the *Mystic Light* CD to brighten your aura. Doing *Triple Mantra* daily is a way of cutting out the negativity so that it cannot enter your life. Negativity behaves like a germ. And those germs are always there, but our antibodies protect us. The practice of mantra is a protective source. Working with the Word is a self-protective device against all animosity known and unknown. It is a simple science. The use of the Word is a timeless, simple truth that allows you to gracefully face the challenges of time and space. This, the greatest power of man, is completely at your disposal. As you absorb our Divine Spiritual Wisdom, your consciousness expands, and you are filled with so much light that you become unshakable. Above all, in this age, the way of the heart will prevail. To begin the day, use your first waking breath each morning to utter the phrase, "I Am, I Am." For now is the perfect time to learn this Divine Spiritual Wisdom and serve the planet. As the light of love, truth, and justice streams down toward the earth via the pentagram, we must realize how interconnected we all are.

The time has come for us to align ourselves with a new level of spiritual consciousness. We may only reawaken our awareness of our spirituality and divinity if we become dedicated to our personal growth and development. The jewel of our spirituality may only be uncovered through self-mastery, self-knowledge and self-realization. The successful Kabbalist and Yogi acquires these skills in several stages through positive manifestation, through thought, selfless behavior, and generosity of spirit at all times. Once reserved for the few who were set apart from the rest of humanity and were specially trained with rigorous and demanding discipline, the pursuit of spiritual mastery is now available to all those who seek. Universal Kabbalah creates a methodology that cuts to the essentials of the work, eliminating all of the unnecessary ideological and semantic adornments and encumbrances with which they were clothed in the past. The quest remains the same, but the technology for accomplishing it is far more precise and accelerated in its design.

Universal Kabbalah is a spiritual discipline that alters, transforms and expands human consciousness in order to give birth to a spiritual consciousness that is introspective in nature with the sole aim of serving the divine in all fellow beings. This method of study also guides the student to higher states of consciousness by providing a philosophy of life and an ethic to organize and structure daily life so as to provoke higher incarnations of consciousness within the current life cycle. This transformation and expansion of one's consciousness can be pursued simultaneously through our Self Study course, and a willingness to examine one's character on a continual basis. By practicing with the Word, it will inspire you, it will make you strong, it will carry you through any adversity. You will possess applied consciousness, depth and strength, wisdom and intelligence as well as intuition so that you may be flexible and adjustable. The practice of the Word will bestow upon you a state of consciousness of self-confidence, self-equilibrium, and self-balance, leading to radiance. There is an exact science, an exact technology, an exact knowledge which allows a human to manifest the most high in the essence he wants. By meditating on the power of the Supreme Being, mankind can experience direct connection with His Spirit and the unseen realm; the angels of the great God will surround you, imparting unimaginable celestial treasures and the spiritual knowledge of all natural things.

We believe in the power and efficacy of the Word which went forth at the creation of the world, and which is now "lost" to the majority of humans. That Word is supreme. Since the fall of man, it has become our only hope. By practicing with the Word humans can get to infinity without interpretation or understanding. The Word has the power to create that consciousness in us. And our sacred wisdom helps man to regain this LOST Word of divine and terrestrial authority. As we grow inwardly, we gradually find this Word as it pertains to our mission in life. And the Word of God is what opens the heart of the ignorant man to Godhood. The practice of the word or mantric way leads to the process of regeneration, which is the spiritual birth that results from the marriage of the consciousness, the emotions and the intellect. The regenerated soul is a purely spiritual offspring of the marriage, within each individual, of the spirit and body. True regeneration, then, acts on both the spiritual and physical vehicles in awakening and renewing the soul powers. It causes right speaking, thinking and acting, thereby renewing the cells and tissues of the physical body, raising them to a higher state of vibration so that they are better able to coordinate their functions with the spiritual vehicle. As previously alluded to, when we consider that regeneration is the process of renewing, recreating and reproducing latent soul powers from a part of the complete individual by the action of the spiritual vehicle of man, we come to understand that regeneration actually reproduces a new organism from a portion of the complete individual.

The mantric way, then, prepares men properly for the worship of God in spirit and in truth. It is the science of rebinding man with God that brings about the accomplishment of beneficial changes in our fundamental state of being. These changes then allow us to become the servants of the universe or agents of God who bring those who are guided by their heads and led by the turbulence of passion to the ways of peace, light, and wisdom.

The acquiring of the Word leads to action—to good and necessary works for the benefit and upliftment of humankind and the glory of God. The mantric way leads to *action* in the name of the unknowable Divine Being; and its effects are magical, in that they rest upon the marvelous, innate spiritual powers of mankind. Our practice is built upon the mystery of the Word, which is the link between our energy and the divine energy, for the Word is love that flows; it is a divine shield that protects you. By practicing with the Word, you hear the Word from which you can get the lost Word, the light of lights. It is the light of lights because it is the essence of enlightenment. When you repeat the Word, you invoke the original divine intention of that Word. As soon as this Word rises in your own heart, you touch God, you touch perfection, and then you begin to understand the divine tongue, and the secret that was closed for so long seems to be revealed. Whoever you are, whatever you are, wherever you are, in speaking the Word, you humble yourself before your creator and seek his blessing so that Wisdom may flow through you. The simplicity of this path is not in ritualism, but in the reality of practicing with the Word, so that the one who has no hope can have hope; the one who has no virtue can have virtue; the one who has no grace can have grace. If we are ever mindful of our humility and thankfulness that the creator has seen fit to preserve these divine teachings and offer them to us through the masters who have held and hold these teachings in sacred trust, our hearts will open and we will be filled with the sweetness of divine love. If you cannot open your heart, work with our Divine Spiritual Wisdom and ask Heaven to help you, so that you may bring the luminous beings into your life. The Word is the linking bridge between the finite and Infinite consciousness, leading you to a stage of grace, greatness, fulfillment and achievement.

Only the true opening of the heart may show us how to genuinely connect with all beings seen and unseen, giving us mastery over the element of air, and bestowing upon us the sight to perceive all spirits that cannot be seen by the naked eye, and the gentle command over these beings who are always around us. When we open our heart through practicing the proper use of the Word, and live fully from the heart, these beautiful beings become helpful friends and messengers of God. The single element we must possess is that of faith; for the Word saves us from the trap of time. If we earnestly practice and master the Word, we may cross the ocean of the time cycle with complete ease, circumventing all obstacles and contacting luminous and helpful beings most people would never consider even existed. We increase our faith through chanting prayer, the ultimate power; that power lives in us and waits for us to call upon it to bless our lives. When you master the Word the sound of your voice becomes alive and healing. From the voice you can find out the true growth of a person. You do not need to see the them; just hearing his/her voice will tell you exactly how evolved he/she is. In other words, the level of spiritual growth of a person is evident in their voice. The practice of chanting mantra brings out the healing aspect of one's voice. Mantra is not only a code projection to decode the mystery of divinity, but also the mantric science is the principal structure of protection and happiness.

It is essential that as we move through the jungle of life, we equip ourselves with the protective power of the Word, for there is no greater refuge. A stream of divine power runs through those who practice with the Word. When the practice of the Word is combined with study of the Divine Spiritual Wisdom, you arrive at a place of knowledge and understanding where nothing can hurt you. The Word is God. Vibrate the Word and let the Hand of God protect you, and His supreme divinity direct you. Use the Word, and let the majesty of God's omnipotence sustain and protect you. Vibrate the Word so that the eternal goodness of God may lead you, as His boundless charity inflames you. The hand of God has brought us the divine destiny of which we speak, and vigorous souls have adopted a human body in order to walk into it. Our divine spiritual technology is a system that prevents man from becoming bogged down by the limitations of environment and circumstance, the strain of indignity and depression, the sorrow of calamity and cruelty, and the pain of betrayal and treachery. Through the Divine Spiritual Wisdom, we see that human independence grants us the right to be and function as a direct descendant of Almighty God. With the seeds of the Divine Spiritual Wisdom sown in many lands and across the boundaries of man-made divisions, it has taken root in the hearts of many people and shall sprout gloriously. Wherever our breath vibrates, so too shall its wisdom. Wherever we walk, it shall precede us with the authority of heaven, establishing jurisdiction so that our future generations can prosper and live in grace. Our goal is to carry the Divine Spiritual Wisdom to all four corners of the globe. Then, humankind shall recognize that the greatness of God is beyond the boundaries of space, and imperial human dignity will be established. All shall live together in peace, tranquillity, understanding, and happiness. When the true Yogi and Kabbalist experience the indescribable power of the Word, he realizes that the true mystical experience is beyond description, and cannot be explained to one who has not experienced it himself. For all the one who has merged with the Sun of Suns can do is pass on the divine spiritual science so that the worthy can open the heavenly gates which are sealed to the unworthy. The divine bliss caused by the ecstatic experience of the true opening of the heart leaves one speechless. All one can say is, "Lord your loving kindness is better than life. Through the Word my lips shall joyfully praise you. I will bless you while I live. I will lift up my hands in your name.

My soul shall be satisfied." Let the hand of God be your help and rejoice in the shadow of His wings. It is only by practicing with the Word that the Lord can stretch His hand down from above and deliver you from the tides of karma and negative forces. Then you will blossom like a well-nurtured flower, for you are protected by the Lord who made Heaven and Earth, the Keeper of truth, the Executor of justice. Practice chanting prayer and praise Him like His angels, like the Sun, the Moon, and the shining stars for He is the heaven of heavens. Praise the name of God, the Great Architect of the Universe. It is His alone that must be exalted.

4

THE FALL OF MAN

THE JUDEO-CHRISTIAN BIBLE relates that at the dawn of creation, God alone dwelled in the pure estate; He originally used a fraction of this immortal substance to create the first man. The indestructible form of Primitive Adam, or Archetypal Man, manifested through the will of the Creator without any physical use of matter, simply through the breath of life. The Archetypal had a spiritual body that was perfect and indestructible. God created this divine emanation and glorious form, in order to fulfill a particular mission, to defeat the rebel Angels who had defied God's law and fallen from Grace. Fascinatingly, the archetypal man enjoyed celestial powers and privileges associated with the first estate. His spiritual body was ideal, his intellect unlimited, the elements responded to his pure thought alone, and his relationship with the Creator was free and unfettered.

God's most important gift to archetypal man was that of free will; the freedom to chose. Yet, Adam and his counterpart Eve, the soul of the universe, chose to misuse their free will; they poisoned their purity and innocence when they chose to eat the forbidden fruit of the Tree of Good and Evil. This error brought about the fall from the pristine spiritual condition of immortality and bliss into the gross physical world. Originally a unified being, man's being was shattered in the fall; his cells became those of the souls of men and women who people the world. Thus, the fallen Adam does not represent an individual man, but rather the sum total of all men and women in their ulterior differentiation.

Man's individual and universal downfall was brought about by a rebel Angel who had fallen from Heaven. The exiled angel lived as an animating principle of matter, which was not yet in existence as realization, but only as a germ of consciousness, like the fruit in the seed or the child in the maternal ovum. He tempted the imagination (called Aisha by Moses) of Adam, presenting a line of reasoning guaranteed to ensure man's expulsion from Heaven.

According to the dark Angel's argument, that which resists and is part of the seen world is more powerful than that which is ideal, invisible and perceptible only to the spirit. Led astray by this idea, Adam imagined the following: if he supplied the principle of matter with the means of transforming from a state of germination to that of reality, he would unite the spiritual power of God with the material power. Since the consequences of this combination were unknown, Adam fancied that he would thus become master of his creator. Once this idea was conceived, Adam and Eve executed it with their free will. When they consumed the forbidden fruit, they united themselves with matter, granting it the principle of existence that it lacked. Immediately, all man's spiritual organs were enveloped in this matter, which he thought he could control as he pleased, and the principle of egoism, rebellion and hatred, which constituted material essence, filled his being and destroyed all his lofty aspirations.

Once they awakened in this universe of matter, the immortal being of the original man and woman withdrew behind the cover of a mortal shield into his/her innermost self. Immortal wisdom sacrificed itself by taking on the cloak of mortality so that its inner power could be preserved deep within man's consciousness and one day potentially raise the mortal once again to the status of immortal.

Thus, original man willfully divided himself from his spiritual essence, submerging his soul, and rendering him susceptible to unhappiness, suffering and death. As soon as he was imprisoned in material form, Adam sank under the elements over which he once reigned. The instant humankind forsook the spiritual fruit that God so lovingly gave them for material fruit from the forbidden tree, he could no longer have unlimited access to God. To this day, man cannot regain his celestial state until he can find his way back to the outer portals of heaven. After the fall, when Adam turned from his inner self, God to his outer self, his own created Satan, he absorbed into his being the possibility of evil, which he was once entrusted to destroy. Evil will only cease to exist through the restoration of man in God.

When Adam fell he lost all goodness and beauty. When man deliberately flouted God's divine law, his indestructible body, a sanctuary of the divine spirit and the true ark of covenant, was destroyed. Wearing the shackles of death, man became the slave of the enemy of evil he was supposed to combat and punish. Thus, deprived of all his rights, and drowning in the bitterness and sorrow of his new circumstances, he no longer dared to show himself to the One who had justly deprived him of his original powers. Formerly the perfect emanation from the breast of the Eternal, man's humiliation was complete. Clothed in a destructible material body, he was forced to suffer under the tyranny of his demonic conqueror, until, filled with sharpest pain of his crime, and moved to repentance, he asked for divine clemency. For having sinned of his own free will, he found the consequences of his actions unbearable and implored his Maker for deliverance. God had to intervene in order to mitigate the consequences of this catastrophe which had materialized Adam and the whole of nature which constitutes his domain.

Before the Fall, human beings had the faculty to perceive and understand the hidden, eternal truths via an inner spiritual organ given to us as a result of our incorruptibility and immortality. Allow yourself to imagine, for a moment, that at this time we were thinking, spiritual beings with glorious, impassive forms. The disordered acts of original man, which influence us, his descendants, altered this state of being. Through his misuse of free will, original man led himself, and us, away from the divine law and covenant by attacking the happy, peaceful realm of eternal unity. In other words, it was the misuse of free will that caused us to be separated from the land of Light. As a consequence, we were given the material form that has been passed on through generations. We became dual in nature, possessing both a gross, terrestrial body and a spiritual, celestial soul. Now, we are no longer intellectual immortal beings, for we have been joined with the destructible, mortal body of matter that is subject to decomposition and death. This is the primary consequence of our separation from Divinity. We have become trapped in a cycle of life and death. Where we once dwelled in the land of Light as the greatest and most powerful of the beings emanated by the eternal, we are now deprived of our sovereignty as pure and perfect beings.

Having rendered ourselves mortal and corruptible, we received the outer organs, referred to as the five senses, which rule us. This envelope of senses is truly a corruptible substance found in our blood, forming the fleshly bonds that bind our immortal spirits and make them the servants of our mortal flesh. This joining of an intelligent spiritual being with a material body was a degrading phenomenon for all spiritual beings. From this imperfect union arose, and continues to arise, all our misfortunes. The part of us that is material and animalistic is reducing us to the condition of the vilest of beasts. We have become slaves to our physical sensations and needs. Indeed, at present, our inner faculty is enveloped in gross matter to the extent that the external eye cannot see into the spiritual realms, we are deaf to the sounds of the metaphysical world, and our speech has been paralyzed so that we can barely stammer the words of sacred import that were once ours and through which we held sway over the elements and the external world.

All mystics agree that once Primitive Adam used his free will to commit this crime against the divine law, this resulted in the materialization of universal man. Now the crestfallen Adamic being was given the skin of a beast with which to clothe his nudity, a symbolic allegory of the history of the fall. From that time forward man was required to refine and purge the lower, animalistic characteristics he added to his nature through suffering, tribulations, and the abandonment of his will into the hand of his creator. Reincarnation was the main instrument by which salvation was to be acquired, and since all men are cells of one and the same being, individual salvation will be complete only when collective salvation is an accomplished fact.

Seeing his once glorious and splendid creation suffering in the most abject misery, God knew that man was feeble and powerless by himself. Subject to all the fluctuations of the planets, man is affected even by the stars, which fire their influences upon him. God sought to mitigate the terrible effects of man's decision by giving him a leader to guide him along the new path which had been made for him. Man's place was taken by another being who elected to do man's work and to lead him back to the perfection of his first state. This being whose symbol is the Star of greater light, is known as IESCHOUAH (*yea-hesh-shoe-wah*), the universal repairer, the mediator between God and man, and the special agent of clemency and mercy. The universal repairer has been sent to shackle the original principle of evil and deliver the children of man from the former enemy of divine unity and perfection.

In other words, after the commission of man's reprehensible crime, the eternal sent an infinitely powerful Repairer to raise man from his disastrous fall and redeem him to his original purpose. This powerful agent Repairer came to manifest his triumphant power over that which was corrupt in the universal temple. To the embarrassment of his enemy, he manifested this power in time, and on behalf of man's descendants, by uniting his divinity with humanity. The Repairer is the most effective divine aid that man can pass on to his descendent. This is accomplished through repentance, an act of grace that must be performed in the name of, and in unity with, the universal reconciliatory agent, the Repairer. But, even though man was supported and strengthened, he could only reach his end through continual combats, in which every effort of his will was needed to triumph.

To help hasten the eventuality of this salvation, the divine Logos, or Word, was sent down to man by God to help man overcome the fear of physical death. Man must work not only for his individual salvation and return to grace, but also for the reintegration of all other created beings. The task of humanity, individually and collectively, is to become re-integrated into the archetype, so that the state of Archetypal Adam may be restored. Until we are re-assimilated, we will continue to suffer the consequences inherent in the physical world, including disease, pain, and death. Our leader is the light of the world himself, Christ, or Ieschoua, the light anointed, the single mediator of the human race, the way, the truth, and the life, the light of ages, the wisdom, the only means by which man can again attain God. Christ, or Ieschoua, the greatest of all envoys, the world savior and universal regenerator, fastened his whole attention on the primal truth, whereby man preserves his existence and can again attain the dignity which he possessed. In the condition of his degradation, he laid the foundation of human redemption. Those who are capable of light are united through spirit and truth.

It is only in the school of light and wisdom that one learns to know God, nature, and man. Here one works quietly for numerous incarnations to reach the highest degree of knowledge, the union of man with pure nature and God. Understand, there is only one God, one visible Sun, one truth, and one way that leads to the great Truth. Whosoever finds this way possesses all wisdom in one book, all power in one power, all beauty in one beauty, all riches in one treasure, and all bliss in one good. The sum of these perfections is the Christ Force, for Christ is wisdom, truth, and love. As wisdom he is the principle of reason and the source of the purest knowledge. As love he is the principle of morality and the essential, pure motive of will. Together, love and wisdom complete the spirit of truth, that inner light that internally illuminates the transcendental subjects and gives them objectivity. God became human in order to make man divine. Heaven united with earth in order to transform earth into Heaven. Christ is the light of the world and within the Christ Force lives the genuine reality, the absolute truth. Each one of us can prove this to ourselves through our own experience, but first we must receive the principle of reason and morality. We must receive Christ as the truth, as wisdom and love. Then, this truth will guide us to our happiness.

5

THE PATTERN OF CREATION: 3-7-12

THE THREE MOTHER LETTERS

The Tree of Life is comprised of ten Sephiroth, distributed along three pillars. The left pillar of Judgment, the right pillar of Mercy, and the central pillar of Mildness or Equilibrium. These three pillars correspond to the three canals of the spinal system known in the Hindu system as, *Ida*, *Pingala*, and *Sushumna*. Interestingly, Sushumna, Ida, and Pingala, correspond to air, water, and fire.

Life cannot manifest on earth, as well as in the human body, without air, water, and fire. The heavens were produced from fire, the earth from water, and the spirit from air; this last element existed as the reconciler between fire and water. Each element corresponds to one of the three mother letters, *Aleph* (air), *Mem* (water), and *Shin* (fire). These mother letters are the determining factors in relation to the spread of the forces of creation, and therefore are the determining factors of all creation. God, then, created a universe that originated with the three mother letters. The same way, we can safely say that the human body is a universe that God in the spine created and continues to recreate from the Sushumna, Ida, and Pingala, or the three mother letters.

Ida and Pingala spiral and crisscross along the length of Sushumna, the central channel in which the kundalini force is at work flowing up and down in order to vivify and set in right motion the chakras and create projections of energy and light. The ladder of bones, represented by the central pillar and Sushumna, and referred to as the spine, is also

THE TREE OF LIFE

1 Ehieh
Kether- The Crown
Metatron
Hayot Ha-Kodesch - Seraphs
Reschit Ha-Galgalim - The first vortex (Neptune)
♆

EQUILIBRIUM

FEMININE-PASSIVE | middle Pillar | MALE-ACTIVE
Left Pillar | Mildness | Right Pillar
Judgement | | Mercy

1 Kether – Crown
2 Chokmah – Wisdom
3 Binah – Understanding
(DAATH)
4 Chesed – Mercy or Love
5 Geburah – Judgement or Severity
6 Tiphareth – Beauty
7 Netzach – Victory
8 Hod – Glory
9 Yesod – Foundation
10 Malkuth – Kingdom

IDA | SUSHUMNA | PINGALA

3 Jehovah
Binah - Understanding
Tsaphkiel
Aralim – Thrones
Chabtaï – Saturn
♄

5 Elohim Gibor
Gebourah - Force
Kamael
Seraphim - Powers
Maadim – Mars
♂

8 Elohim Tsebaot
Hod – Glory
Mikael
Bneï-Elohim – Archangels
Kohav – Mercury
☿

9 Chadoï - El - Haï
Iesod - The Foundation
Gabriel
Kerubim – Angels
Levana – Moon
☽

10 Adonaï - Melek
Malkout - The Kingdom
Sandalfon
Ischim - Perfect Men
Olam Iesodoth - Earth
♁

2 Iah
Hokmah - Wisdom
Raziel
Ophanim - Cherubim
Mazaloth – The Zodiac (Uran...)
♅

4 El
Hesed - Mercy
Tsadkiel
Hachmalim – Dominations
Tsedek – Jupiter
♃

7 Jehovah Tsebaot
Netzach - Victory
Haniel
Elohim – Principalities
Noga – Venus
♀

6 Eloha ve Daath
Tipheret - Beauty
Raphaël
Malahim – Virtues
Chemesch – Sun
☉

called the Serpent, the wand, or the Scepter. It plays an important role in the religious symbolism of the Ancients. The Greeks symbolized the three canals in the *Caduceus*, or Winged Staff of Hermes. This symbol consists of a long rod (the middle pillar and central Sushumna) that ends in a knob (the pons of the Medulla Oblongata). On either side of the knob are arching wings (the two lobes of the cerebrum). Twisted around the length of the staff are a black serpent (the left pillar and Ida) and a white serpent (the right pillar and Pingala). Understand, the *Caduceus* represents man, with all the innate powers and possibilities he must develop in order to manifest Divine power. Each human being, then, is a living *Caduceus*. The central wand is the spine and the two intertwined snakes are the currents that descend from the two hemispheres of the brain. The human spine, with its twenty-six vertebrae, is a special unity with similarities to Divine unity. Like Divine unity, man can manifest his powers through the three, innate canals. This makes man a true divine image and the likeness of the Creator.

God, as the absolute principle of all beings is one in essence, Aleph. God, as manifesting his powers outside Himself through His own faculties is three. The spine or Aleph is a symbolical of one light arising out of three different luminaries, and stand for the principle of unity arising from adversity. The numerical value of Aleph is one. Number one which symbolizes God. It is indivisible, void of all parts, nothing is before one. All things proceed of one into many things. All things endeavor to return to their one, from which they proceeded. One is referred to the most high God who is all seeing. He is Omniscience and Omnipotence. He is one and innumerable, yet creates innumerable things of himself and contains them within himself. One creator who is over all, by all, and in us all. From one man Adam all men proceeded, from that one, all become mortal. From that one through Ieshouah they are regenerated.

Aleph is the first letter of the Hebrew alphabet. Aleph represents the three luminaries. It is the basis of all calculation and all act done in the world. One will find unity nowhere but in Aleph. However, being formed of 2 Yods and 1 Vau it also has he numerical value of 26. Twenty-six is the divine incommunicable name: Yod He Vau He (10+5+6+5 =26). We also have 26 vertebrae in the spine.

This figure 26 is obtained by adding two Yods (10 + 10) to that of Vau (6). The number 26 reduces to 8. Therefore Aleph has three numerical values: 1, 26, and 8. Eight is the number of healing, justice and fullness. Eight, formed of two superimposed spheres (heaven and earth), is the symbol of the all-pervading mind of God.

We can see therefore that the numerical values of Aleph refer to three aspects of the divine:

(a) *One:* its absolute identity.

(b) *Twenty-six:* its latent creative power expressed by the Word.

(c) *Eight:* the universality of God presence in whose mind is all that exists.

The number three represents the three basic principles of all embodiment in their state of simplicity and original inaction. Harmonyum works on the entire body through the One (Aleph), or the spinal column and its twenty-six vertebrae (the divine, incommunicable name—Yod He Va He, has a numerical value of 26 (Yod =10+He=5+Va=6+He=5 = 26). The spine, Aleph, is symbolic of one light arising out of three different luminaries, and stands for the principle of unity arising from adversity. Aleph contains the number twenty-six. In other words, Aleph relates to the structure of the spinal column with the two Yods symbolizing the two currents, Ida and Pingala, which spiral and criss-cross the length of Sushumna which stands for the one Vav, the central channel in which the kundalini energy flows. The wand stands for the masculine principle, the serpent stands for the feminine principle which entwines itself round the masculine principle in order to heighten and intensify its powers.

The central rod represents the mental dimension where as the polarized serpent represents the Astral dimension. Again, we have 26 vertebrae in our spine. Our spine, then, is like God due to the power within it of divine production or emanation. It manifests 18,000 times the quaternary number of divine perfection through the 72,000 nerves attached to it (4 x 18,000 = 72, 000), of which at will, it increases the images around itself by being the body's supply center. That is why the philosophical addition of the number four, produces the number 10, which is the expression of all Divine and spiritual, corporeal and temporal material existence. And by reducing this same number to its roots, you will recognize that all beings originate directly or indirectly from unity.

Therefore, it is through the direct divine emanation of the energy that runs through the visible and invisible spine that we as spiritual beings acquire the future eternity and infinity of our action, even though they may be limited in their effects when we cease to remain attached to the unity of divine action that runs through our spine.

The 72,000 nerves add to the number 9 which is a number of initiation. The number 9 is a combination of the three ternary combinations, the uniting of which is brought by a new work of the life principle which is within them, and constitutes the matter and material bodies in the form assigned to them by the original law which presided over their formation.

It signifies the end of temporal beings, because the form or material bodies is only maintained by the presence of this particular short life, which sustains its existence for the duration prescribed for each species. In this universe everything is life; the smallest grain of sand has its life principle without which it would soon cease to exist, would go back to the invisible reserve of elements from whence it came. This principle of life, as existing separately from the body, with which it is linked, adds its own number to the number 9 of the material body, and it is only by this connection that the individual exists in his individual form; but as soon as the principle of passive and passing life, which kept these parts together, is removed, this body is left to its nonad number, which, without its link, tends rapidly towards its decomposition and eventual dissolution. Then the elements, the principles and the combinations, of which it was made up, successfully return to their source.

The Caduceus of Hermes can also be the Sephirotic Tree of Life with its two lateral pillars of Severity (positive), of Mercy (negative) and the central pillar of Equilibrium. Two currents descend from Kether, pass through Chokmah and Binah, cross at Daath, pass through Chesed and Geburah, cross at Tiphareth, pass through Netzach and Hod, cross at Yesod, which symbolize the generative organs. As we said earlier, in the physical plane the central wand is the spinal column and the two serpents are the two currents, positive and negative, running along each side of the spine (Pingala/White and Ida/Black spiralling around Sushumna).

These currents cross over at the level of the nape of the neck, pass down through the lungs, cross over again at the solar plexus, continue downward through the spleen and liver, cross over again at the level of the navel, pass through the left and right kidneys, cross again at the Hara chakra and finally, pass through the sexual glands of a man or the ovaries of a woman.

The two currents follow a path that criss-crosses over from one side to the other. The first current starts from the right hemisphere of the brain, passes through the left lung and the heart, crosses over to the liver, back to the left kidney and from there, to the right sexual gland and terminates its trajectory in the right leg.

The other current starts from the left hemisphere of the brain, passes through the right lung, crosses over the spleen, back to the right kidney and from there, travels through the left sexual gland to the left leg.

The magic wand is polarized both positively and negatively, by the two snakes which intertwine around it. The two serpents represent the two currents of cosmic life, the current of attraction or love and the current of repulsion or hatred twined around the axis of the world. It is these two currents that move the world and everything in it. All movement is triggered by attraction and repulsion. An initiate who knows how to channel and control these two currents can knowingly attract or repulse other beings.

The Universal Kabbalist uses them to attract light and repulse darkness. To attract Heavenly blessings and repulse the forces of evil. The whole world was created by these three forces. Ida and Pingala are the lunar and solar forces. They correspond to the lower and upper triangles of the Star of David contained in the flag of Israel. They stand for water and fire and are the most fluctuating forces of the elements. Happiness comes from their balance.

The magic wand restores the connection between the higher world and lower world. It connects the two worlds so that the current may flow freely between them. The central powerhouse in the world above produces plenty of current, but if we want our light to burn on earth, they have to be connected to the main current. The magic wand is the connection that makes this possible. Harmonyum works on the locations of the body that are the material representation of this connection. As a result it activates the connection between your head and heart, and the one between your soul and spirit.

By connecting the higher and lower worlds, we are inviting the will of the Father to be done on earth as it is in Heaven. Therefore, a connection is established between our spirit and the Spirit of God, between our soul and the Soul of the universe, between our intellect and the Cosmic Intelligence, between our heart and disinterested Love. Then, our hands and Word start working for us. This takes care of the Atmic, Buddhic, Mental, Astral, and Physical planes. Harmonyum brings your vibrations in harmony with heaven, causing you to be luminous so that the forces of nature can understand and listen to you. As a result they hear and grant your request. In order to bring to earth the purity, light, and harmony from above so that the earth becomes a reflection of heaven—we must make the connection. The power house is in the sublime region of the higher world.

If we want our lamps to light up and function we must plug them into the power line from above. The magic wand is an electrical connection that has to be plugged into Heaven. If your vibration is in harmony with Heaven, the forces of nature will understand and listen to you. They will hear and grant your request. When the connection is established, the current of life produces the most marvelous results.

SEVEN CERVICAL VERTEBRAE

The three mother letters issued forth the seven double letters, each of which embodies the characteristics of one of the seven sacred planets. These seven double letters, representing the seven cervical vertebrae correspond to the seven Archangels in charge of the seven planets which are the seven mighty expressions of spiritual truth. The angelic rulers of the seven periods manifest just as distinctively and as perfectly through the seven periods of the yearly cycle, as in the greater cycle of our consciousness. Through planetary forces and the differentiation of the signs through which the planets pass, each double letter manifests in the universal scheme. It is significant that the seven letters are double, as it indicates the dual nature of the influence of the seven sacred planets; each has both positive and challenging aspects. Similarly, each of the double letters has both a hard and soft aspect to their sound. Choosing the hard or soft aspect modifies the meaning of the words in which a given letter appears.

Finally, like the seven planets, the seven double letters represent the seven Elohim, expressed through the seven nature notes and the seven colors into which the one white light (or the Yod) is broken up. We must realize that each soul who is born is an emanation from the Great Spiritual Being that rules the universe. This is referred to in the Bible as the Elohim, or the Seven Angels of the presence, which rules the signs of the zodiac through the planets. Each of the seven planets are ruled by an Archangel that brings upon the soul varying experiences, joys, temptations, and tests, which a careful study of the greater map of the heavens will elucidate and make clear. From the beginning of time, this great clock of heaven has marked off its hours, and planetary rulers—the regents of the stars—have passed in grand procession with the torch of their inimitable illumination through the pathway marked out.

There are seven avenues through which the Sun of righteousness, the incarnate Word, can shine forth and illuminate the hearts and minds of all classes and conditions of humanity. They represent the seven gates to the new Jerusalem, that inner temple of truth in which each type of humanity (disciple) can receive the illumination of the inner mysteries, face to face and heart to heart through his own special avenues of thought and teachings. The inner shrine is where the One light reveals those inner truths which cannot be given directly to the uncomprehended multitude, but which are the basis of the outer light shining forth from every true disciple of the Christ force. Jesus Christ fed the multitude with five loaves and two small fish, and with the remaining fragments he gathered twelve baskets full. The seven cervical vertebrae stand for the forces of five exoteric planets and the two esoteric planets hidden behind the Sun and the Moon. These seven planetary forces must be recognized and assimilated, so that one can fill the baskets with the forces of those planets expressed through the twelve thoracic vertebrae and symbolized by the twelve signs of the zodiac. The planetary rulers of the seven sacred powers, or Creative Forces of the Cosmos, govern the kingdoms of the macrocosm and manifest in the twelve divisions of the celestial zodiac.

TWELVE THORACIC VERTEBRAE

One can transpose the name of God twelve different ways to find the twelve banners of the mighty name that correspond to the twelve signs of the zodiac. They are IHVH, IHHV, IVHH, HVHI, HVIH, HHIV, VHHI, VIHH, VHIH, HIHV, HIVH, HHVI. The twelve thoracic vertebrae represent the twelve simple letters, which are associated with the twelve signs of the zodiac. The twelve zodiac are all represented by animals, it has been said that man receives the forces of his animal nature from the zodiac. This is quite true, for in man's body can be found traces of all the lower kingdoms which he has unconsciously raised to a higher scale simply because they have been built into the human body. Yet through the planets he receives the higher forces by which to transmute the lower. Humans must take all the forces of the animal kingdom which he finds within himself and lift them above the mere animal and transmute them into perfected powers of the higher self. These letters represent the twelve properties and potencies that form the earth's aura. As the planets pass through the zodiac, various potencies that are specific to each sign awaken and blend with the force of the respective sign's ruling planet to send forth its own particular planetary cocktail, or force, whose influence we feel on planet earth. These distinct forces act in concert to help earth express all the possible manifestations available to her. In other words, the earth must assimilate the potency of these forces so that she may unfold the perfect pattern she is destined to express in her evolution. Alchemically, number 12 pertains to the great work. The great work is before all things the creation of man himself. It is the full and entire conquest of his faculties and his future. There are three major operations in the Great Work. The first is the transmutation of all base forces and passion in ourselves into spiritual Gold, thus setting the soul free from all prejudice and vice. It is called the transmutation of all base metal into Gold. The second is the creation of the universal medicine which cures all diseases; and third is the production of the philosopher's stone which turns everything it touches to Gold. This work is related to twelve, because only as man gathers the forces of the twelve signs of the zodiac and builds them into his life can he become a Magus, one capable of completing the Great Work.

Also, the elements composing the human body are carbon, oxygen and hydrogen, together with twelve mineral salts which stand for the twelve thoracic vertebrae, along with the sign of the zodiac as follows:

1. Potassium phosphate with Aries and the brain.
2. Sodium sulfate with Taurus and the elimination of water.
3. Potassium chloride with Gemini and the animal tissues.
4. Calcium fluoride with Cancer, the teeth and the elastic fiber.
5. Magnesium phosphate with Leo and the nerve sheaths.
6. Potassium sulfate with Virgo and oil, hair and nails.
7. Sodium phosphate with Libra and the acids
8. Calcium sulfate with Scorpio and tissue cleansing.
9. Silica, called the surgeon of the system, with Sagittarius.
10. Calcium phosphate with Capricorn and the Bones.
11. Sodium chloride with Aquarius and the control of water.
12. Ferrum phosphate with Pisces, the blood and vital energy.

The Great Work is spoken as an operation of the Sun because in nature it is the subtle force of the Sun, which transmutes all gross seemingly dead things into new life, as the delicate flower arises from the decomposing humus. Within man's body the spiritual Sun must accomplish the same great work. The number twelve expresses the entire scheme of manifested creation. The Sun, the Moon, the Earth, and all the stars of heaven, with the rulers thereof, each has its appointed place and definite work to do in bringing into physical manifestation and completion the Grand Plan. Through it the Great Law (the Lord God) of divine love and wisdom may bring forth and perfect Man made in his image. It pertains to the complete expression or fruition of the divine trinity within the circle of its manifestation. Twelve is called the number of fruition or the manifested universe. By the fourfold expression of the divinity, the triangle. Four is the number of mundane manifestation.

6

THE NATURE OF MAN

MODERN MAN EXISTS as a combination of opposing natures. Where Man was once a thinking, spiritual being with a glorious, impassive form, after the Fall we were merged with a material body subject to decomposition and death; a merger that all spiritual beings experienced as a horrific phenomenon for it revealed, and continues to reveal, the vast contrast between man's will and divine law. Now comprised of both imperishable, metaphysical, transcendental substance and material, perishable substance, we have become the battleground for good and evil. The nobility and grandeur of our origin shines forth via the intellectual and the immortal aspect of our being, while our propensity to indulge in physical sensations, needs, and pleasures derives from our material forms. This combination of the limitless possibilities of the human mind with the limitations of the human body creates uneasiness. While the body of man, susceptible to infirmity and destruction, drags itself over the Earth, the mind of man soars, taking in the entirety of the universe yet frustrated by the material shackles that prevent it from truly probing the depths. It must be stressed that this combination of great faculties and few means was not the intention of the Creator. Rather, the intention of the Creator was that Primitive Adam should maintain the glorious form he was given, the one suitable for manifesting the activities of his spiritual strength.

Even though humankind has fallen from great heights, God, who created all things in order that they may be submitted unto the will of

Man, has included humankind in His project to bring His works to perfection by making Man participate in His Divine and Terrestrial work. God has, in fact, made the whole earth and its inhabitants subject to him. Moreover, God has given humankind the means by which he may work with the many spirits that preside over manifold realms through God's bidding, thereby allowing man to profit from the good fortune and happiness these divine spirits may impart. Some of these celestial creatures govern the archangelic world, and others the angelic world. Some regulate the motion of the stars, while others offer direct assistance to humankind. Finally, some continually sing the praises of God. In addition, there exist both spirits who correspond to the planets and elemental spirits. The planetary spirits are Saturnian, Jupiterian, Martian, Solar, Venusian, Mercurian and Lunarian spirits, while the spirits of the elementals exist in fire, air, and water. The elemental spirits, in particular, happily serve those who learn how to respect their nature and for whom they have an affinity. In order to work with the divine spirits, and garner material and spiritual prosperity through their benevolent assistance, man must understand how to work with the invisible realm.

It cannot be stressed enough that the crude bodies in which we find ourselves are not the true organs of investigative power. As it stands now, human beings are living in exile, deprived of our true essence and real powers, for the imperishable remains enclosed within the perishable. Due to a desire to know and subject everything to his will, humankind analyzes and dissects, attempting to uncover the sustaining principles of land, sea, and heaven. But, these efforts are futile because our level of knowing has been reduced to that which we can perceive via the five senses. Because our fragile material organs do not allow us to probe beyond perceptible forms, our search for knowledge only scratches the surface of corporeal beings and the activity of secondary agents.

The story of the Fall resonates with each of us because it is applicable to every soul. Incarnation itself represents the first, individual fall, and everyone in the human family has inherited the sinful nature Primitive Adam adopted when he neglected his inner self in favor of his external self, in effect creating his own Satan. Understand that this world is not our true home. This is the reason happiness eludes us. The purpose of our Earthly journey is to free ourselves from the shackles of physicality and material obsession so that we may be restored to the condition that was originally ours. Indeed, resistance or submission of the incarnate soul to the passions of the physical plane will either destroy or constitute a second fall. Man, as the descendant of Primitive Adam, is called upon to refine and purge the lower qualities of his nature via suffering, resignation in the face of trial, and turning over his will to his Creator. Salvation and restoration to grace, or reintegration, is the goal. Reincarnation is the primary means of salvation. Because we are all cells of Primitive Adam, it is imperative that we understand that our individual salvation is directly linked to our collective salvation. We are aided in both our individual and collective salvation by our Divine Spiritual Wisdom, which gives us a particular interpretation of Creation, the Hierarchy of Beings, the Fall of Man, and the way for Man to return to his original estate, thereby regaining his original privileges. The Mantric and Inner Way of Reintegration, which rests on the power of the divine Word, transmits the mysterious spiritual power.

A new universe is presently birthing, bringing to earth, as well as every particle of existence, every parallel universe, and every life form in this and other realms, a high vibrational energy. As we approach the time when the veil of illusion that cloaks the world is lifted to reveal the realm of light, wisdom, and love, the faculty of animal man will be progressively removed so that man can appear in his original purity. This process is causing a battle between light and darkness, between the head and the heart, because animal man is struggling against the coming of the spiritual man. A level of separateness and a dispersal of consciousness heretofore non-existent on Earth is occurring. As a result, people are experiencing the mental, emotional, and/or physical stress that can affect relationships with friends, loved ones, and one's self.

As we have discussed, all human misery is born from the corruptible material of mortality. However, we must never lose sight of the fact that the immortal, incorruptible principle still exists within our inner being. When this principle is developed to the point where it is able, as it were, to devour that which is corruptible and mortal, man can be freed from misery. We must regenerate in order to loosen the corruptible matter that keeps our immortal being bound in chains, and the active power asleep. When this is accomplished, we can experience a rebirth in which the spirit of wisdom and love rule, and the animal nature that keeps us slaves to the physical obeys. Such rebirth establishes the conditions whereby we are able to enter into communication with the world of higher intelligences. It is to this end that we have been given the gift of the human form, for it is only within the human form that the Soul can realize God and retrace the footsteps of its descent in order to reach its original home. It is through the physical form that man can manifest the actions of his intellect and will.

Our limitations result from our separation from God, the supreme principle of Good that is the true light and only support of creation. It is only in God that there is harmony and perfect accord among all beings. Understand that God created the world in which we live for a purpose. Part of that purpose is for us to have an environment where we can learn certain lessons via the type of punishment and spiritual privation we suffer. Through the long process of evolution of the selfhood, our soul personality learns these lessons and draws ever nearer to our spiritual principle. The purpose and desire of our entire earthly existence, then, is to re-enter our innermost state of Heaven where the only real and true thing is God's light. Our destiny is to overcome the struggles we face in the material world so that through our own efforts, our own proper use of free will, we may regain our early and original state. Indeed, it is through freedom of thought and action that we may return to God via the path of tribulation that leads to knowledge, the knowledge that leads to wisdom, and the wisdom that leads to eternal truths. We must never forget that in addition to our material body we still possess an immaterial body that is glorious and perfect. We can no longer afford to have our souls slumber, shackled to that which holds them down. It is time for our souls, our segment of the eternal soul of the universe, to work with our sacred science so that it may unfold in the wisdom of the ages and, in so doing, prove us worthy of expanded comprehension of our parent soul. We must release our souls by turning our sights to God. This will allow us to unfold in the glory of our own divinity.

Through our immaterial bodies, we may once again enjoy all the rights of immortality. Therefore, we must strive to re-awaken the interior faculty of our immortal spiritual body so that the grandeur and nobility of our pure origin may shine forth. It is only by having the courage to open our hearts and awaken our souls that we prove that we are worthy of our divine inheritance. It is only by truly opening the heart that we earn the right to ascend into consciousness.

It is through the power of the Word that the angels come to your aid. The striking difference between man and all other beings in nature is demonstrated in his speech and voice. This is due to the eternal truth, "In the beginning was the word…" In man, the Word expresses itself through speech. Speech, the language of the mind and our spiritual faculties, is in us. Our speech contains all of our strength and energy, even if we are not outwardly expressive. It is the means by which we communicate with all the beings of nature, and with God through prayer. Lastly, it is the means by which we must become the law of the universe. Do not confuse the active power of speech with the passive sounds made by animals. Amongst all the beings that inhabit the Earth, we are the only ones who are endowed with the full power of speech and, therefore, the Word. Remember, that as the image of God, we have been empowered through the Word to make ourselves heard by the whole of nature and raise ourselves to the throne of the eternal. You must never abuse this privilege, however, by asking for negative outcomes, for cursed are those who will use the name of God in vain and employ for evil purposes the knowledge and good wherewith He has enriched us.

God has also assigned a guiding, protective spirit, a *genii*, to each human being. A genii watches over and preserves the individual to which it has been assigned. Elemental beings such as ourselves, the genii are more able to render service to us when we become aware of their existence and the rules that govern them. When we open our third eye, we can experience direct contact with our genii.

Within every human being there is a spiritual body. Via that spiritual body, we acquire knowledge of the higher worlds. These higher worlds, the worlds of soul and spirit, are just as real as the world we see with our physical eyes and touch with our physical hands. The blind cannot lead the blind. One can only receive guidance as to how to go about awakening the advanced powers of spiritual perception by those who already possess them. The method of safe awakening is exact. And you will find it in our sacred science. Moreover, those who have been initiated into the nature of the Divine Spiritual Wisdom know that only those who have been experientially exposed to it can truly gain understanding. Spiritual wisdom is not something acquired through casual spiritual window-shopping. Rather, the Divine Spiritual Wisdom will find you under all circumstances if you provide the universe with proof of your earnest and worthy desire to attain this higher knowledge in order to heal yourself, uplift others, and serve humankind.

Within each of us lies a holy place. God is already sitting in you. Your breath has been given to you as a sacred gift. Use it to make your mind as pure as and lighter than air, and your heart warm with heavenly joy. Rise beyond religious boundaries to find the spirituality within. Without spirituality, we experience social chaos. With true spirituality, we can control our minds. When you clean your holy, internal temple, Light and Love pour into you so that they can then pour from you. The following meditation, Sodarchan Chakra Kriya, is one of the greatest meditations you can practice, for it has considerable transformational powers and the ability to retrain the mind.

Meditation: Sodarchan Chakra Kriya

POSITION:
Sit in easy pose with light neck lock, chin slightly pulled in (Jalandhar Bandh). The eyes are fixed at the tip of the nose.

MUDRA:
The left hand is in Gyan Mudra, thumb to index fingertip, resting on the left knee. The right hand uses the thumb and index (Jupiter) finger or little (Mercury) finger to block off the alternate nostrils.

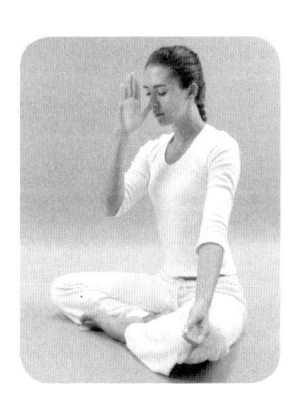

MANTRA:
Wahe Guru (pronounced *Wha-hey Guroo*)

BREATH:
Block off your right nostril with your right thumb. The other fingers are straight and pointed up. Breathe in through your left nostril and relax your left hand on your left knee. As you hold your breath, mentally chant *Wahe Guru* 16 times. Pull in your navel point as follows: once on *Wha*, once on *Hey* and once on *Guru*, for all 16 repetitions (for a total of 48 pumps). Then block off your left nostril with your right index finger and exhale slowly and deeply through your right nostril. Continue.

TIME:
Continue for 11-31 minutes. Master practitioners may extend this practice, first to 62 minutes, then to 1 1/2 hours per day. If you are a beginner, you can start with 3 minutes and gradually build to 7, then 11 minutes and so on.

To end, inhale, hold the breath 5-15 seconds, exhale. Stretch the arms up and shake every part of your body for 1 minute.

COMMENTS:

Sodarchan Chakra Kriya opens all the chakras, thereby giving you a special energy. It goes all the way to the brain and rejuvenates it by giving an additional amount of megawatts to your neurons. The personal identity is rebuilt, giving the individual a new perspective on the Self. It can purify your past karma and the subconscious impulses that may block you from fulfilling your highest potential. It balances all the 27 facets of life and mental projection, and gives you the pranic power of health and healing. It establishes inner happiness and a state of flow and ecstasy in life. It opens your inner universe to relate, co-create and complete the external universe.

To gain these benefits requires different efforts from different people. Each mind has stored up its own pile of negative thought and energy, so each pit is cleaned on its own time and scale. You decide how much time you have and you need to invest in this practice.

Sodarchan Chakra Kriya can remove impressions of past male partners in the female's arc line. Furthermore, a recently published medical study showed it to be more effective than antidepressant medication in treating psychological issues. Eleven minutes a day will build your confidence and capacity to know who you are; 31 minutes a day will give you great strength and discipline. One year will make you feel fantastic; 1,000 days of doing this meditation and no one will be able to match your strength. It helps inner happiness and ecstasy in life. It gives you a new start, against all odds. When external pressure becomes too great, it brings power from the inside.

"There is not time, no place, no space and no condition attached to this mantra. Each garbage pit has its own time to clear. If you are going to clean your own garbage, you can clean it as fast as you can, or as slowly as you want."

7

THE AGE OF THE CHRISTOS

At different points in human history, the Heavens have undertaken the task of repositioning themselves in order to awaken human beings from their evolutionary stupor and bring them closer to God. We are reaching a time when the great clock of Heaven is ticking toward a most important era. Our solar system is now entering the Golden Age. This Age is the sign of the son of Man in heaven, referred to in the New Testament as the time of the New Dispensation or Age. The Age of Aquarius is ruled by Uranus, which is the higher vibration of the planet Venus. Uranus is the planet of individuation and Universal Consciousness gained through sharing and love. During this Age, all that has been hidden must be made known. This is the most important of the sub-races of the Fifth Great Human Race inasmuch as we are now planting the seed of and preparing for the Sixth Great Human Race.

The first race of humankind, or the Lemurian, was in reality the first physical race. When its final hour of dissolution came, the whole continent of Lemuria, sunk beneath the waves and with it the Race disappeared. As the Racial hours passed by, a certain embryonic imprint was deposited in the soul of humanity, in the thought world, and in the astral realms so as to be developed and built in the subsequent Races. We are now entering the sixth sub-race of the Fifth Great Human Race. There is a very important relationship between the Third Race, which was the first race to materialize from the mere astral bodies, into the denser material bodies and the Sixth Race, which is the third hour it completed the triune manifestation. In the spiral of evolution the Sixth Race stands directly over the Third Race; it completes the triangle. It is the other diagonal side. The lower, more dense, physical, horizontal line of the triangle is represented by the Fourth and Fifth Race.

At these times of transition, the universal karmic clock sounds the alarm indicating that all is not right with the world. The last four times this occurred, civilization did not heed the alarm. As a consequence, these civilizations were destroyed. Presently, we have arrived at the moment in history when the fifth change is taking place. The world is beginning to change back to its primordial state of spirituality, and the flaming sword is removing itself from its place between man and the Tree of Life. In other words, falsehood, false rules, and dogma are being destroyed in order to permit the Spirit to be sensed and felt in actual life.

We are living in the time that has long been prophesied as the Last Days. Indeed, the wars and natural disasters taking place in the world today have already been prophesied. These occurrences are not about the destruction of the planet, but rather the bringing about of a new, great cycle of humanity. Before this cycle can come to fruition, the earth and humanity must undergo a natural process of purification and preparation.

From now until the year 2012, we will collectively experience a cosmic shift heralded by a time of intense conflict as the cosmic forces fight for dominance and the Earth fights for survival. The world will go through years of purification, a sort of planetary near-death experience, via natural catastrophes and/or warfare as the old world is laid low so that a new world of spiritual, collective consciousness with universal love at its core can be built. The world will experience a period known as the "Flood," the "Descent of the Clouds," or the "Rising of Aphrodite." We are currently in a terminal station for a 25,000 year period. The years that lead to 2012 are called "The Descent of the Clouds." During this difficult transitional time, great and lasting changes will occur in the global landscape. There are certain signs that can disclose to you the nature of the descent of the Cloud. When you open your eyes fully, you can plainly see that the world is in a state of chaos. Many nations are ravaged by war and disease. Natural catastrophes and weather irregularities are making headlines. Many people are living in states of pain, confusion and poor health. We are inundated with technologies that speed up the pace of our lives to unnatural levels.

Indeed, we have come to regard the Internet as indispensable to our professional and personal lives. Interestingly, *www*, the prefix to all websites, is the equivalent of 666 otherwise known as the number of the beast. When 666 is reduced we arrive at 18, the number of the tarot card the Moon. Eighteen represents a materialism that strives to destroy the spiritual side of nature, a materialism that uses divisive and/or deceptive tactics to gain position and/or wealth. Eighteen also warns of treachery and deception from known and unknown persons, friends and enemies. In the extreme, the number 18 is also associated with wars, social upheaval and revolution. Under the energies of 18, everything conspires to destroy the native. Hostile spirits, represented by the wolf, are laying traps, while servile spirits, represented by the dog, hide their treason behind a mask of flattery, and idle spirits, represented by the crab, gaze upon the ruin of the native without concern. What's worse; the native is often ignorant of such conspiracies. Therefore, one must be on guard. He must watch, listen and act accordingly.

Conversely, in the Jewish tradition, 18 is regarded as a positive number that brings blessings. It is derived from the word *Chai*, which means Life. The word *Chai* is made from *Chet* and *Yod*, and together they make 18. Our science of spiritual numerology also reveals that the name of Christ, which stands for truth and light, adds up to 18 as well. This further demonstrates the positive aspect of this number. Moreover, the Bij mantra *Sat Nam*, which means "Truth is my identity," reduces to 18. Therefore, with the advent of the Internet nothing can remain hidden. All truth shall come into the light. There is no way around it. The Internet, then, plays two roles, that of the beast and that of the angel. Therefore, depending on the ways in which you choose to use it, you will either develop the beast in you or strengthen your angelic side.

As we further explore the energies of the number 18, we see that it can be reduced to 9. Nine is the number of Mars. The energy of Mars rules over construction as well as destruction. It also rules the energy of sex. Once again, when we look clearly and neutrally at the occurrences on our planet, we can see that both the mass media and the Internet are currently riddled with subtle and overt images/messages of violence and sexuality. Indeed, the prevalence of sexuality and violence in the content of traditional and non-traditional media outlets depicts the unbalanced energy of Mars at work. The pendulum has swung to the extreme and these forces, long held in check by social custom, ethics, modesty, cultural law, physiological ignorance, and ecclesiastical restriction, are rapidly being released into the global scene.

The open nature of the Internet has made it fertile ground for many avenues of expression. However, this has also made it a playground for depravity and sexual deviance providing a haven for those who traffic in darkness and prey on the unsuspecting. These unchecked, rampant forces can represent a serious danger for children, and for people who turn to the Internet to unknowingly fill the void of emptiness in their hearts and souls. Some places on the Internet have even become the invisible bar or nightclub, the place where one can go unseen and unregulated, to fulfill the low animal desires, the beast in humankind.

Burying oneself in endless surfing on the Internet or spending hours in other on-line activities, can remove one from the healthy, positive, life affirming relationships with others and one's self. Rather than experiencing the joy and sorrows of life in real time, people have retreated into the shadows. Such loss, such emptiness, builds on itself. One can soon find themselves completely isolated from the heart essence of life. For some individuals, the Internet has become a substitute for human interaction and connection. And for others, such use has become an addiction, a destructive tool to escape the realm of the heart where personal issues are resolved and love flows forth. This addiction is no different from others in that it becomes a slippery slope that leads the addict down a path of pain and destruction. Children are particularly vulnerable when it comes to the Internet with its wealth of knowledge, games and activities at their fingertips. In some cases they stumble onto violent and sexually explicit sites that shape their tender minds in negative ways, and in the worst-case scenario, are drawn into harm's way. It is imperative that we nurture our children by providing them with activities that strengthen their character, intellect, emotional intelligence and spiritual awareness.

These precious hearts and minds will be our spiritual, community, and political leaders, as well as our hope for tomorrow.

During the years that lead to 2012, these unimpeded and dangerous forces will provide ample evidence of Nature's powerful forces and elements of destruction. Do not despair, however, for in due time these energies will give way to their more balanced aspect, and with it, a more peaceful and healing way of life will be initiated.

To reiterate, the Internet is ruled by the Moon archetype and the planet Mars. Not only does the Internet have its dark side as discussed above, the Internet also has the immense capacity to positively serve humanity in several ways through our conscious use. Just as it is a powerful tool used to promote messages/images of sexuality and violence, it can also be an equally, if not a more powerful tool, when used to promote messages/images of truth, justice and peace. We can counteract the dangerous misuse of the Internet by using it to universally disseminate uplifting information to the masses. Indeed, when the gentle message of Love is backed by the energy of Mars, it is extremely powerful. Such messages can open a multitude of doors and overcome many obstacles. Therefore it must be stressed that when used consciously, the Internet can become an integral tool for spreading the message of Love, Peace, and Light throughout the planet, thereby uplifting humanity.

In addition, the political map will be altered. There may even be a change in the geophysical stability of the world. Sacrifice, including loss of life, will be a necessary part of this process. In short, the new Age cannot emerge without sacrifice and transformation. Individual and collective karmic debts must be paid in full. As the Truth of Life descends from the world of Eternal Light to illuminate the minds, regenerate the hearts, and renew the souls of the sons and daughters of the light, those who harmonize with the rhythm of the coming Age of Aquarius will form the seedbed from which a new global culture and consciousness develops. Therefore, the human race is currently experiencing the descent of what is spiritually known as the "new Jerusalem," or the "new city of peace." The new Jerusalem symbolizes the advanced civilization, know as the Golden Age, which will be ruled by the King of Peace through his representatives, the Masters of the Divine Spiritual Wisdom. The Aquarian

Age, the Age of the Christos, is the Era of the feminine principle, for the Christ force manifests the feminine qualities of love, compassion, and intuitive intelligence. These qualities exist in, and can be expressed by, both women and men. As it descends from heaven, the new Jerusalem must find the proper conditions for its physical manifestation.

In addition to changes in climate and the physical condition of the earth, there will also be a change in human thoughts, feelings, and relationships. While change is often painful and accompanied by disaster, clinging to faith in the divine will help us understand the law of cycles and shows us that disasters, whether global or personal, are nothing but the adjusting process of the law of justice.

Therefore, the time has come for human beings to work with the Christ force to be granted an open heart and the high consciousness necessary for humanity to be spared from the ravages of the four elements—air, fire, water, and earth—and to live in harmony with the entire universe. It is important to realize that different types of disasters are caused by a disturbance in a given element. For example, a disturbance in the air element, which corresponds to the heart center in humans, leads to cyclones, storms, tempests, whirlwinds, tornadoes, and hurricanes. A disturbance in the fire element, which is caused by a misuse of money, power and control causes car accidents, explosions, wild fires, and burning. A disturbance in the water element, which is caused by a misuse of sexuality leads to storms, tidal waves, cloudbursts, hurricanes, drowning, and accidents at sea. (Water dangers can also involve a disturbance in the air element.) Finally, a disturbance in the earth element, which corresponds to insecurity and all forms of addiction, such as drugs, alcohol and smoking, leads to landslides and earthquakes. Work with the Divine Spiritual Wisdom contained in Universal Kabbalah and pray that nature, especially the works of man, be spared the ravages of air and fire, and that humanity be spared the calamities of water and earth.

Global change begins with personal change. In order to successfully negotiate these challenging times, we must learn the sacred science of Divine Spiritual Wisdom. So, learn these sacred teachings and show your worth and trustworthiness to yourself, others, and the entire universe. Let the reputation that precedes you be of the highest caliber. Again, the world needs you now. Don't let global consciousness down. The role of Universal Kabbalah is to impart this wisdom to those who seek it, helping initiates to transform themselves into a living and healing Star of David. Once you begin to be open to Universal Kabbalah, a channel of beatific knowledge and blessings reveals itself to you in all its sublimity. This divine wisdom creates a spiritual wedding, also known as the *Mysterium Conjunctionis of the Alchemists*, within you. As a result, man, who is lost in the ocean of Being without a true sense of his role in the universe, is transported to the confines of Omneity where he realizes his relationship and relatedness with God. He learns to recognize the greater presence and power that is God, is reminded of his true origin and the blueprint of his life's plan, and is shown where he will return at the hour of his death and his true identity, including the infinite and loving omnipresence and might of our creator. When he accomplishes even a fraction of this task, he becomes a pure channel of love, peace and light to all. Blessings continuously flow into the life of such a person, whose nature has been transformed by this sweet and incomprehensible merger with the Will and Mercy of the Lord. In other words, this beautiful and sacred wisdom, through the mystical marriage of the lamb, causes spirit to spiritualize matter and turns a human into pure spiritual Gold.

Working with our sacred science will align you with Heaven, creating deep healing and an understanding of the unifying divine force that is inherent in every aspect of creation. Those who learn Universal Kabbalah are students of the Divine Spiritual Wisdom that teaches life mastery. By learning this sacred science, attuning to the Cosmic, and living in harmony with natural and spiritual laws, you are able to invoke cosmic aid in all your endeavors. Moreover, you will be assisted in regaining your lost inner powers so that you are able to operate from your Universal Mind. The Divine Spiritual Wisdom that flows from Universal Kabbalah, then, improves the quality of one's life, restores one's health, solves the many problems of one's existence, and ultimately leads to happiness. The ability to affect such positive changes is what makes it authentic. Your challenge during this transitional time is to work with Universal Kabbalah so that you may become deeply attuned to cosmic processes. Learn the Divine Spiritual Wisdom and expand your experience of both self and life. As we commence with the rough ride ahead, use the Divine Spiritual Wisdom as your seat belt and your parasympathetic nervous system for damage control. The Divine Spiritual Wisdom will give you the right attitude, help you see these coming years from the right angle, and turn even your most painful experiences into blessings. Rest assured in the knowledge that its practice is the fulfillment of the divine union with the children of the light that will bring about the Golden Age that follows this transitional period.

As falseness and darkness have seeped into the world's arts, sciences, religions, and political systems, even the wisest among us may have difficulty discovering and walking the path of truth and light. Many believe that if they acquire financial security they will survive this difficult period of transition. They are fooling themselves. All great men of wealth and power have ultimately lost the game. In his coffin, Alexander the Great used his last breath to say: *Place my hands outside so the world may see I have conquered the world, but I have not taken anything with me.* The problem we face during this time of evolution stems from a limited definition of self and reality. The problem is not how to reinforce external security in the world, but how to attain internal security through spirituality. The only way to feel comfortable in this Age is to learn the Divine Spiritual Wisdom and practice with the Word so as to experience your vastness. The only effective method of releasing your insecurities is to develop a relationship with your soul. The challenge of life is to face ourselves and our life lessons with grace, while learning the sacred science in order to experience our true selves and the universe. Every tragedy, insult, injury, and betrayal is a wake-up call that gives us the opportunity to learn the sacred science, practice with the Word, and serve humankind. You can change your destiny, which is written on your forehead, as soon as you commit to learning the Divine Spiritual Wisdom, practicing the Word, and serving others. When you are meditatively graceful and serve others, you are protected by the Hand of God; you attract His creativity and divinity. As a result, you do not fall short. Your consciousness, knowledge, and understanding; your body, mind, and spirit; your past, present and future, are all balanced. Decide that you will learn the Divine Spiritual Wisdom and serve others, and remember that regardless of what happens, if you maintain your grace, God will always be with you. If you are a graceful human being, and serve others, the entire Prakirti, all the Creativity of God, will come to you. Your grace and service to others will attract the entire divinity of God to you. And all the prosperity, beauty, bounty, bliss and happiness, will come to you.

Yet and still, many will be unable to successfully deal with their lives as the tides of this Age continue to change and we move closer to the year 2012. They will be thrust into the dark labyrinth of depression, dissatisfaction, and lack of purpose that lies at the core of their hearts. Indeed, increasing numbers of people will suffer from the devastating afflictions of acute depression, weariness, and fear. As mankind collectively experiences the evolution of these conditions, some will fall into the void of insanity. Even those who resist this level of darkness will still seek release in the form of escape, expression, and/or suicide, as the Age of the Glory of Self forces them to take a hard look at themselves and see who they truly are. There is a side to all that follows the light, the shadow of which we must endure. It is this shadow, the shadow of the self, that will strike with a vicious intensity. This shadow, of course, is a teacher who brings the opportunity for growth and self-realization. People thus afflicted, however, will desperately need guidance in order to be uplifted to a state of mind that is relaxed and calm. Understand that the technology and methodology or the scientist and traditional medical practitioner, even armed as they are with much research and preparation, will fail those in distress.

As those who walk the path of the Divine Spiritual Wisdom, it is both our responsibility and joy to share it with others, especially those in dire need. To serve others, you must have power. Therefore, do not hesitate to learn this sacred science, for the world is in need of this knowledge. When others reach out to you, touch their hearts with your smile, your touch, and the sweetness of your word. Go directly to the light in others by seeing God in all and serving God in all. In this way, you will allow others to be who they truly are, stripped of the illusions and limitations that hold them in captivity. In other words, strive always to enhance the core essence of power, purity, and piety in yourself and others. Keep in mind that you may feel that those in need of help are bombarding you. Prepare yourself for the rush by fortifying yourself. If you learn our sacred science and practice with the Word, you will have the capacity to receive and serve others by sharing the healing tools you have acquired. As this knowledge ripples outward to touch many, the world will come to understand that peace, tranquility, divinity, grace, and living in ecstasy is the true way. The relationship between God and man will be perfected and never again be subject to collapse.

While individuals, groups, and nations will be confronted with suffering, the rise of the Divine Spiritual Wisdom will generate great reforms. As a great flood of divine spiritual light washes over the Earth, the suffering of humankind will be alleviated. Moreover, the falsehood and darkness we have been, and will be, subjected to shall be forever removed so that a single standard of truth, available to all, may be established. Our Divine Spiritual Wisdom enables you to direct your life through the power of the Word, so as to root out and cut off bad karma. As a result, you become neutralized and free to understand the aspect of Infinity. Infinity is not something that confines you. The Divine Spiritual Wisdom is the science that allows you to survive this Earth and beyond, for one must be released from the Earth's magnetic field so that they can be liberated. It cannot be stressed enough: *Learning the Divine Spiritual Wisdom and working with the Word is the ultimate weapon against disease, fate, bad karma, evil forces, and destructive habits.* The more you tune in with the Divine Spiritual Wisdom, the better off you will be. You will develop a vast, beautiful aura and your positive influence will be felt far and wide. Learning the Divine Spiritual Wisdom and working with the Word will grant you the capacity to attune yourself to the various energies and flows of beneficial force and states of consciousness, as well as the beings of light that provide guidance and understanding. Moreover, the Word creates and synchronizes the essence, and its practice is a qualifying factor in enhancing your intuitive intelligence. It gives you a very powerful meditative mind, and control of your frontal lobe. Control of the frontal lobe grants control of the personality.

CALLING UPON THE CHRIST FORCE

We must invoke the help and protection of the Christ force and allow the great architect of the universe to look favorably upon us. Christ which is the Word made flesh, means anointed one, Messiah, anointed by the light of God. The Word, the Logos, is the second aspect of the trinity. In the trinity of Brahma, Vishnu, and Shiva, Christ corresponds to the incarnation of Vishnu, the preserver, the God-Man dispeller of Darkness. Christ consciousness is an unlimited form of consciousness. It is the consciousness or awareness of the self in and as the Christ, and an attainment of the balanced action of the power, wisdom, and love of the Father, Son, and Holy Spirit as well as the purity of the Mother principle within the heart. In short, Christ consciousness is faith perfected in the desire to do the Lord's will; hope in the salvation of Christ, Jesus by the path of his righteousness performed in us; charity's excellence in its purest love of giving and receiving in the Lord. Attaining this level of consciousness is commensurate with attaining the level of consciousness that was realized by Avatars such as Jesus, the Christ. In other words, realizing Christ consciousness means a realization within the soul of that mind which was in Christ, Jesus. The Christ Self, then, is the individualized focus of the only begotten of the Father, full of grace and truth, the mediator between a man and his God. It is our own personal teacher, or master, who officiates as high priest before the alter of the Holy of Holies of the invisible temple made without hands and located in the heart of every human being. The Universal Christ individualized is the true identity of the soul, the real self of every man, woman, and child to which the soul must rise.

Filium Dei unigenitum,
Et ex Patre natum ante omnia saecula.
Deum de Deo, lumen de lumine,
Deum verum de Deo vero.
Genitum, non factum,
consubstantialem Patri:
per quem omnia facta sunt.
Qui propter nostram salutem
descendit de caelis.

Only begotten Son of God,
Begotten of his Father before all worlds.
God of God, light of light,
Very God of very God.
Begotten, not made,
being of one substance with the Father:
by whom all things were made.
Who for us men and for our salvation
came down from heaven.

By invoking the Christ force, we are working with the Lord of Heaven, the Lord of the throne of miracles, the Master of the invisible world. This always brings reality, love and heavenly royalty into our actions. If there is no heavenly royalty in us, our reality will never be with us. You are working with the Christ force, the Lord of the community of light. The Christ force is everywhere, throughout all of creation, and is the healer of all creation. It comes from the Greater Light, that same Light that gives light to the entire universe. It cannot be bound by one religion, country, or house, for it is the force that calmly grants its healing to everyone. The Christ force heals with purity, restoring those in pain and strengthening those in need, as purity is its nature. Regardless of whether you are a Christian, Jew, Muslim, Hindu, or Buddhist, the Christ force will help you when invoked. Never turning its back on those who invoke it, the Christ force even quietly heals those who deny its very existence. Again, the Christ force is timeless, spaceless, creedless, genderless, colorless, and classless, and therefore not beholden to the influence of one particular person or group.

Understand, there is only one God, one visible Sun, one truth, and one way that leads to the great Truth. Whosoever finds this way possesses all wisdom in one book, all power in one power, all beauty in one beauty, all riches in one treasure, and all bliss in one good. The sum of these perfections is the Christ force, for Christ is Wisdom, Truth, and Love. As Wisdom he is the principle of reason and the source of the purest knowledge. As Love he is the principle of morality and the essential, pure motive of will. Together, Love and Wisdom complete the spirit of

Truth, that inner light that internally illuminates the transcendental subjects and gives them objectivity. God became human in order to make man divine. Heaven united with earth in order to transform earth into Heaven. Christ is the Light of the world and within the Christ force lives the genuine reality, the absolute truth. Each one of us can prove this to ourselves through our own experience, but first we must receive the principle of reason and morality. We must receive Christ as the Truth, as Wisdom, and Love. Then, this Truth will guide us to our happiness. Christ is the Active, Intelligent Cause, the Great Chief and Guide to whom the order of the universe has been committed until a time when man, now in a state of separation, has been reconciled with the One and only Source. This universal order was originally entrusted to humankind before the fall. Now, we are under Christ's aegis until we regain our rightful place in the universe.

We follow the Christic path, believing in the immortality of the soul and in its final reintegration. Universal Kabbalists pray, and apply the precepts of Christ in their daily lives. We love others with neutrality with no expectation that the love will be returned. We participate actively to share the Divine Spiritual Wisdom to help lighten the burdens of others, and awaken the love of the great Architect of the Universe in their hearts. For He is the One giving us will, strength and power to face the challenges of time and space gracefully. Humans think God is in the head, when in fact he is hidden in the heart of the simplest man. To be a servant of the universe, one needs to be humble, simple like a little child, charitable, loving towards your neighbor, and forgiving of your enemies. It is imperative for us to realize that our individual and collective mission is to bring all the talents and virtues of Heaven that have been sown in us into full bloom. We are meant to live the life of our spiritual soul, and must strive to do so. There is no joy equal to the joy of learning and working with the Divine Spiritual Wisdom. Once you have tasted the sweetness that is your birthright, you will want for nothing else.

Universal Kabbalah leads to Christic consciousness. It shows the way to illumination. It gives you the blessings of happiness and health while on earth. It gives you that pure energy which activates the inner faculty of the spiritual and incorruptible body, putting you in direct contact with the higher world, and all things start to work automatically. Nothing will properly work in your life until you activate this interior faculty of your immortal body. It moves the energy from your Silver cord to your Gold cord and you get Superconsciousness in Consciousness. Our lineage descends from Adam to Noah, from Noah to Melchisedek, and on to Abraham, Moses, Saul, David, Solomon, Zerubbabel, and Christ. It is only in the school of light and wisdom that one learns to know God, nature, and man. Our sacred teachings originate with the Creator himself, and have been perpetuated since the days of Adam.

When you invoke the Christ force, you invoke the creative power of the universe, the manifestation of the healing power of the Sun, the God, the Ultimate, the Infinite. Through the grace and blessing of the Word made flesh, that dwelt among us, and we beheld his glory, the glory of the only begotten son of the Father, full of grace and truth. This is the only pure reflection in creation of God the Father who dwells in you as a Bio-metaphysical physician, and it is He who works with the lifeforce of a person, and is guided by the innate intelligence of that person, to do what is right. The Christ force is the symbol of the Great divine mystery of the manifested Godhead, and the healing universal law of manifestation, so mathematically correct and precise in every detail, that it displays an expression of a fundamental infinite truth, the manifestation of God in His works.

Working with the Christ force attracts the beneficial energy of the Star of Great Light into your life, leading to a positive and healing transformation. It brings you knowingly to the unknown, demystifying it so that it then becomes known to you. The moment the Christ force brings you awareness, you start living in the heart and Karma ceases to exist, for where there is heart, there is no Karma. Karma is created when you live outside your heart. Working with *Lumen de Lumine* is a surefire way to follow the way of the heart. In order to accept the Christic energy into your heart, however, you must first create, and then build, a resistance to negative thinking, negative feeling, negative speech, negative action, and negative behavior. You do this by raising your energy and bringing it into harmony with the cosmic laws through the practice of the Word, and living a life of service. In so doing, you will be following the path of high and good work as well as Christ consciousness, and your energy will continue to be transformed.

Therefore if your personality, your identity, and your mental self do not represent the Christ force, you will never know the reality of love and healing. As Universal Kabbalists we have the throne of healing. We have a majestic destiny as the apostles of Christ to bring healing to humankind. The Christ force is the crown of the universe. The planetary Christ is the house of the Lord of miracles and healing. Through the agency of the Christ force we give a little push to the life force of a person for healing to take place. When a person achieves the fullness of soul identification with the Christ Self, he is called the Christed or Anointed One, The Son of God. The Son of God is seen shining through the son of man.

By serving the Christ force, you become the Christ. In order to become a perfect channel for the Christ force, however, you must light the seven candles within, beginning with the one located in your heart. The law of cosmic consciousness exists to create the creativity of the Creator and to present the presence of the Creator. Everyone who has been created can transform that creative energy and blossom into a flower that demonstrates the presence of the Christ energy. Through the law of cosmic consciousness, the Christ force uses the human heart as a transformer. When the high Solar energy, known to advanced initiates as the Christic force, goes through the power of the heart and starts flowing through us, we have a connection with the energy that is no longer unknown to us.

Open your heart. Keeping it closed will only make you unhappy, nervous, and fearful. Meditating on *Lumen de Lumine* and working with the Christ force will prove to be exceptionally beneficial in this age, for it is a practice that will open your heart, causing that soul fire of mystery to transmute your mental and physical consciousness, bringing you into a closer and more perfect union with the Godhead. The seed atom of the soul is in a static or dormant condition and requires the application of spiritual fire, in this case from the sun's ray, so that its static condition can be transformed into one of kinetic activity and its sprout begin to put forth. *Lumen de Lumine* is an expression of the kinetic activity or active burning of the spiritual Sun. Through the flame of divine love it lights the spark in the hearts of men so that the dormant Christ force may be turned into kinetic activity, and the Christ seed in their hearts may begin to sprout.

Listening to *Lumen de Lumine* brings the Christ force into your heart. You can then invoke it to make decisions or to help in your healing work. *Lumen de Lumine* surrounds you with Light, and Light brings youth. The more Light we receive, the closer we are to God. The more sacred fire we have, the more our love is strong. The more divine force we have, the more we are assured that we are on the right path in life. Above all, remember that you must love everyone. Do not hurt anyone's feelings, and always forgive other people's mistakes and weaknesses. As you know, He always stressed that blessed are those who make peace, help those in need, and heal those who are sick. Therefore, open the doors of your heart and bring the Christ force in. Make your heart a place of worship, and it will bring you healing and happiness, for the Christ force will sit within you. With the Christ force firmly planted within your heart, the healing that is occurring internally will heal those around you as well. In other words, you will spread Christic healing to anything in your presence, and contribute to healing the earth upon which you walk. We are all created in the image of God, and therefore destined for Oneness and perfection in God.

8

THE STAR OF GREAT LIGHT

IN ACCORDANCE WITH THE GLOBAL SHIFT in consciousness that is currently taking place, the Heavens drew two pentagrams in October 2004, in such a way that they have rendered themselves neutral. This means that we, as human beings, will not be under their protection again until the year 2012. The pentagram, or five-pointed star, is one such symbol of immense power used by Kabbalists. The great Kabbalist Eliphas Levi called the pentagram the symbol of total power of the mind. Moreover, he stated, the pentagram expresses the mind domination over the elements. It is the star of the Magi, the burning star of the Gnostic schools. All symbols of the gnosis, all figures of spirituality, all Kabbalistic keys of prophecy are resumed in the sign of the pentagram. It is the sign of absolute and universal synthesis. If you stand upright with outstretched arms, you will take the classic form of the pentagram as portrayed by Leonardo Da Vinci's painting, "Vitruvian Man". In this instance, the top point signifies the head, the intelligence that governs the rest of the body expressed as arms and legs by the four lower points. Whether you view the planetary configuration as a star or a human form, the overall symbolism of the pentagram illustrates that a Higher Consciousness reigns over the world of matter. The pentagram represents a reaching toward the Higher Self or the beginning of the Great Work. We are now entering the predicted time, which will bring with it the cleansing of all karma and global enlightenment. Normally, the Heavens and Earth control karma but when the Heavens are neutral, the capacity for tremendous spiritual growth will become available. Therefore, until the year 2012, you have the opportunity to open your heart, so as to re-write your destiny for positive, divine, and spiritual purposes. Now is the time when the Heavens are bestowing the opportunity for personal resurrection. In other words, up until the year 2012 you will be able to cleanse your karma and get rid of all your darkness. This time will create drastic change in everyone's life. And change creates great fear and anxiety. We are fast approaching the time when the veil of illusion that cloaks the world will be lifted. As it is lifted, the realm of light, wisdom, and love will be revealed. Indeed, a new universe is presently birthing, bringing with it a high vibrational energy not only to earth, but to every particle of existence, every parallel universe, and every life form in this realm and others. The faculty of animal man is being progressively removed so that man can appear in his original purity. Everywhere we see evidence of the battle between light and darkness, between the head and the heart, as animal man struggles against the coming of the spiritual man. This is causing a separateness and dispersal of consciousness that has never before existed on earth. As a result, people are experiencing the mental, emotional, and/or physical stress that can affect relationships with friends, loved ones, and oneself.

The world is beginning to change back to its primordial state of spirituality, and the flaming sword is removing itself from its place between man and the Tree of Life. The Truth of Life will descend from the world of Eternal Light to illuminate the minds, regenerate the hearts, and renew the souls of the sons and daughters of the light who are destined to constitute the nucleus of a new humanity. Indeed, those who harmonize with the rhythm of the coming Age of Aquarius will form the seedbed from which a new global culture and consciousness develops. The Word of the living God is beginning to be heard, and it will transform everything. Therefore, for us to feel comfortable, the immortal principal within must expand and absorb the corruptible principle without, so that the envelope of the senses may be lifted, for us to appear in our pristine purity. This process is achieved through a true opening of the heart, via the mantric way, and the development of the internal organ that allows us to receive God. Upon completion of the process whereby we open our hearts and develop our internal spiritual organ, the metaphysical and incorruptible principle comes to rule over the terrestrial principle and human beings, filled with the light of heaven, begin to experience the grace and joy from above. The time has come for us to activate the inner organ of our spiritual body and, in our ascent, develop certain powers that differ from those developed during our descent. The time has come for us to activate our lost interior organ so that we can merge with the absolute in order to bring about internal reintegration. These sacred teachings, along with the luminous beings that have passed them down, are there to assist all ready seekers of good heart, pure intent, and honest motivation. One must understand that this priceless science cannot be learned via your intellect. One need an open heart to penetrate the heart of holy wisdom.

The pentagram represents a balance of the five elements: earth, air, fire, water, and ether. The top point of the star, Spirit, presides over the four lower points, and stands for the soul personality referred to as the Quintessence, or fifth element. Each alchemical element encompasses a phase of our being. Earth symbolizes the body, physical and non-physical. Water symbolizes consciousness of the objective and the subjective. Fire symbolizes our higher and lower emotions. Air symbolizes the material and transcendent intellect. Taken as a whole, then, the pentagram represents mastery of the soul essence over the four elements of man's being through the trials of life. Together, the four lower points of the pentagram represent the essence of the human, earthly experience, as well as how the various circumstances of life must be felt, understood, and ultimately transcended in order for each of us to attain a grounded realization of the divine genius that exists within. The presence of the October 1st pentagram indicates that the time has come when we can no longer deny the internal presence of God in us through the breath of life and our psyches. Of further interest and significance is the fact that the archetypes associated with each of the planets constituting the October 1st pentagram serve to reaffirm the spiritual meaning of the five-pointed star that we will explore in this next section of our discussion.

The pentagram or Star of Great Light, contains the totality of the Christic mysteries. It would be impossible to convey the true Christic mysteries to humankind in our present state. In truth, God and Nature do not seek to present their children with mysteries. Such mysteries are the result of our own weaknesses. Our natures are not, as yet, able to support and bear the chaste light of unveiled truth. Therefore, a cloud or veil, has been placed before the higher world. To be sure, it is a cloud of divine mercy, for in our depleted state of being, the pure light of the higher world would harm us. The mystery is unveiled when we achieve mastery. Indeed, where there is mastery, mystery no longer exists.

The Divine Spiritual Wisdom represents the eternal truths at the core of the Christic mysteries that describe the differences between fallen and regenerated man. These eternal truths are known to the fully realized man, through regeneration, or inner transformation. In order to achieve knowing, however, the heart must lead the way and the head must conform to its plan. Understand that the average man, who is ruled by the head and the lower centers, cannot partake of the mysteries of God. In fact, by walking this path of error he distances himself from God. To experience the mysteries, a complete change must take place in our being. It is the mantric way that leads man to the transformation, re-birth, and interior life of union with God by opening the inner organ that allows us to experience the mysteries. In other words, the mantric way outlines a process of redemption based on an experiential understanding and realization of eternal truths and, therefore, the Mysteries, and is necessary for the ultimate salvation of mankind.

If everyone could bear the look of truth, and the number of good, heart-centered people were greater, then more secrets could be revealed because we would not have to worry about misuse. The fact is those who search with an honest, open heart need only read but one word, one sentence of this sacred wisdom, in order to feel at home and join in these teachings of the heart, these heavenly teachings.

Remember, however, that this work and particularly the coming paragraphs should not be read lightly. It should be studied and worked with. The unraveling of various secrets requires a certain amount of divine, spiritual, and physical knowledge. If you have trouble understanding any aspect of this sacred wisdom, do not dismiss it, simply put it aside for later study, or in this case continue to the next paragraph. Eventually it will become clear.

Now let's delve a little deeper into why working with the "I Am, I Am" or the "Ieschoua" energy found on the *Sounds of the Ether* CD, is particularly relevant to the time ahead. All of humanity operates upon the basic formula of creation, *Yod Heh Vav Heh*, meaning fire, water, air, and earth. *Yod Heh Vav Heh* refers not simply to the Jehovah of the old testament, but also to the basic forces in action of the Ain Soph, the Infinite. This is the pathway, or method of evolution, by which average men slowly progress from human to divine. The elect of light, however, take another path, which is represented by the formula, *Yod Heh Shin Vav Heh*. The pentagram, symbolic of Ieschoua, is formed by the Hebrew letters of the Tetragrammaton, the four letters signifying material creation, interjected by the holy letter, *Shin*. The holy letter *Shin* is a symbol of the Holy Spirit, known as *Ruach Elohim*. This name *Yod Heh Shin Vav Heh* or the spelling IHShVH which is the spiritual spelling of the name, Yeheshuah, or Jesus, gives the formula by which the agent of light performs the great work of spiritual fusion. Fusion, reconciliation, and union are the keys to countering the effects of the Fall of Man so that we may experience reintegration. Now *Yod He Vav He* represents *Adam Kadmon*, man in his integral synthesis, representing a fruitful union of the Universal Spirit and the Universal Soul. To divide that word is to suggest a disintegration of its unity. The letter Shin, Arcanum 21 or 0 in the Tarot, reunites the two fragments, representing the generative and subtle fire, the vehicle for non-differentiated life.

Moreover, *Shin* signifies the Universal Plastic Mediator whose charge is to bring about incarnations that allow the spirit to descend into matter. The letter *Shin*, then, in its role as a sort of hyphen between the other parts of the mutilated tetragram, becomes a symbol of both fragmentation and fixation. Finally, *Shin* also begets the quinary, or number of destruction, when added to the verbal quaternary in the way we have just said. In this respect, *Shin* is the Word, or Logos, the *Yod He Vav He* that incarnates and becomes the suffering Christ, or corporeal man, until such time when he enters into his glory assuring his regenerated human nature.

In other words, *Shin* is given the attribution of fire, and by another mathematical process, it becomes the symbol of the holy spirit. Tradition sponsors the insertion of this letter into the middle of the four-letter Name, splitting it apart, thus forming *Yod He Shin Vav He*, the pentagrammaton or five-letter name. This combination of letters represents the illumination of the elemental or present man by the descent and impact of the holy spirit. As thus formed the name represents the God-Man, symbolized in Christianity by the Christ descending on the man Jesus. The Chief of all agents of light, The Christ, was the combination of all the specialized perfections of the divine agents, of the ancient alliance, into one. He bestowed the touch of perfect unity that opened a new door and destroyed the number of the slavery of humanity. This Chief Agent of all, this savior of the world and universal regenerator, turned man's attention to the primitive truth that allows him to preserve his existence and recover his former dignity. In the condition of his degradation, he laid the foundation of human redemption. Jesus, in this symbolism, represents the natural man who, by devotion and meditation and the theurgic process, opened his human nature to the brilliant descent of the light. It is the enlightenment that all men are destined to enjoy at some far distant time in human evolution. It is this that separates animal man from the God-man, the goal of all mysticism. All mystical techniques, including those of the Kabbalah, represent a method of hastening the slow tedious process of human evolution so that the states of consciousness that we are told will ultimately occur routinely in mankind may dawn today.

Only one planet shows us a perfect geometrical form. The form is pentagonal, and the planet is Venus. Creating five equally spaced alignments over a period of 8 years, her orbit draws the perfect, hidden, and secret symbol of the five-pointed star—the pentagram—in the heavens. Revered by the Ancients as the endless knot, the pentagram is a geometrical form that encodes the Golden Proportion or Golden Cut. The most pleasing of harmonic divisions, the Golden Proportion is the harmonic ratio that the God-Mind sees fit to encode in so many of It's creations. The pentagram indicates the manifestations of light and life, and a potential bond with God. It is a symbol of the Logos—the word made flesh, the eternal spirit, and the four elements under the divine providence of the letters of the name Ieschoua. The four lower points of the pentagram, symbolic of the four elements, are crowned and completed by the fifth element of Spirit, the Quintessence. Making the pentagram calls upon the spirit to descend and infuse the four elements, earth, water, fire, and air. Therefore, it is said that the pentagram connects the intrinsic Divinity within the self with the Divine Self, the wholeness of the consciousness that gave us life, known as God.

The pentagram represents the fiery, purifying, and enlivening power of the Divine that can pierce and bind all negativity, separate the pure from the impure, bring visions, catalyze the experience of higher love, unity, and healing, and even open and close gates.

Some refer to it as the Blazing Star or the Star of the Magi, and equate it with the Star of Bethlehem. Just as the Star of Bethlehem announced the birth of the baby Jesus, the appearance of the Quintiles in the sky heralds the birth of the Divine Christ Child within each and every one of us. This is due to the fact that the pentagram is the embodiment of the Pentagrammaton, the five-lettered name of God associated with the coming of the Cosmic Christ, symbolized by the descent of the divinity of the Christ (the Dove) into the world of matter. The pentagram, then, is the symbol of the heavenly or realized man—the Adam Kadmon, the Divine Prototype, the Angelic Human known as the Atziluthic or Archetypal man in Kabbalistic terms.

The pentagram, the geometry of the Quintiles, is emblematic of the Christ force that is the perfected, concentrated force of the One God, with its procreative power. This same Christ Force resides within each of us. Waiting silently and patiently, it never leaves nor forsakes us. Rather, it sustains us through all of life's circumstances, both good and bad.

Known as Ieschoua, the Christ force is recognized by Kabbalists as being among the hierarchy of supreme forces of the universe. It is the equilibrating, compensating, healing, redeeming, purifying factor of the universe; the light anointed, the single mediator of the human race, the light of the ages, the wisdom, the way, the truth, and the life, and the only means by which man can, once again, attain God. In other words, the Christ Force is the light within that leads to the light without. The greatest of all envoys, the world savior and universal regenerator; the principle of being and of life within us that cannot perish, the Christ force lets us know that the regeneration of our virtues is possible. It tells us that we can ascend to become a demonstration of the Active and Invisible Principle from which the universe derives its existence and its Laws.

In Western tradition the Tiphareth symbolizes the Christ force, or Ieschoua. The Tiphareth is the central Sephirah of the ten holy Sephiroth of the Kabbalistic Tree of Life. He who is filled with the spirit of service to God is filled with the spirit of the meaning of the mystical name, IHShVH (Ieschoua). This name, which we usually translate as Jesus, is also the name of Joshua, who succeeded Moses as the leader of the Israelites. It is the Christ force, Ieschoua, which should be invoked in every operation of psychic self-defense where any human element, incarnate or disincarnate, is concerned. Conversely, when non-human elements, such as elemental thought forms or the Qlippoth must be dealt with, it is the power of God the Father, as Creator of the universe, which should be invoked, with His supremacy over all the kingdoms of nature, visible and invisible, being affirmed. God the Holy Ghost is the force that is employed in initiations, and it should not be invoked during times of psychic difficulty, as its influence will tend to intensify the condition and render the veil even thinner.

When you want to protect yourself, invoke the Christ force or use the symbol of the pentagram of light. It will cause your five tattvas to stand as a shield. Whenever the five tattvas are in pure combination, the seven chakras plus the aura work in absolute harmony. The symbol of the pentagram put the five tattvas into harmony and puts the seven chakras into action, so that our divine, spiritual and physical energies can be put together into a natural and neutral reality, so our chakras can be encircled by the tattvas.

9

TRUTH

What we now call truth is merely relative truth. The spiritual organ necessary for the realization of absolute truth was closed as a consequence of the Fall. Now, the gross matter of our material bodies serves to obstruct our inner eyes so that we cannot perceive the beauty of the higher world. This same matter obstructs our inner ears so that we cannot perceive the sound of the metaphysical world. It also paralyzes our inner tongue so that we are no longer able to utter the powerful word of the spirit, which we not only once pronounced, but through which we controlled outer nature and the elements. While we have come to rely on our five senses for learning, understand that they are composed of disproportionately formed, corruptible substance. Therefore, they are only capable of receiving the semblance of light and the reflection of truth. Corporeal man will not find absolute truth in the realm of appearance nor via the five senses. In other words, truth is not found via external searching in the material world, because truth is not found on Earth. Rather, truth exists within us and we exist within it. We are inextricably linked to the truth, and cannot be separated from it.

Only Christ is wisdom, love, and truth. As wisdom He is the principle of reason, the source of the purest knowledge. As love He is the principle of morality, the essential pure motive of will. Together, love and wisdom complete the spirit of truth, the inner light that illuminates in us the transcendental subjects and gives them objectivity. In order to advance to this level of perception, and experience a realization of higher truth, an organized spiritual body and internal spiritual organ responsive to the reception of light must be nurtured. The spiritual body is founded on an incorruptible, transcendental, metaphysical essence, and we can have no realization of higher truth without opening our inner spiritual faculty. Indeed, the spiritual world and absolute truth exist solely for the inner man, the spiritual man, who has his own inner sensorial system which functions in intuitive and psychic impressions, and allows for the reception of the absolute truth of the transcendental and invisible world. Only the spiritual man is able to use his inner spiritual faculty in much the same way that visible man uses the exterior five senses. As previously indicated, however, in most men this organ lies subsumed under the weight of the sense faculties. Unless we purify ourselves through service, and make the spiritual organs a part of ourselves, we will remain unfit to see, hear, and speak in the spiritual world. We will not experience rebirth. However, once the inner spiritual organ is opened properly, life is experienced as a positive, working flow.

The aim of any spiritual practice is to help the destiny of man through a union with God in spirit and truth. The foundation of Divine Spiritual Wisdom is Truth through the Word. First was the Word, and last is the Word. The Word was the beginning of creation and, therefore, the Word opens the mysteries of creation and helps us communicate with the higher worlds. Our centers of intuition, inspiration, and evolution are all touched by the sacred Word. Truth through the Word is only for those who are sincere and committed, however. The Truth is not available to those who would abuse it, for a sharp sword in the hand of a child can produce fatal consequences. In order to be worthy of Truth, you must rise above greed, pride, and conceit. Moreover, when the universe rewards you with power, you must demonstrate that you are not only worthy of the blessing bestowed, but willing to continue to perfect your human nature. This is achieved by increasing the level of humility, understanding, and compassion that inform your words and deeds.

Understand that all men are called. In turn, the called may be chosen. But, in order to be chosen, the called must prepare to enter. In other words, anyone can look for the entrance to the higher Worlds, and anyone who is within can teach another to seek, but only he who is fit can arrive inside. Those who are ready are linked to the golden chain of light. Interestingly, this often occurs at a point in our lives when we know nothing, and at an unlikely place. Those who seek wisdom should, therefore, seek to become ready. Readiness is achieved by developing humility and the willingness to serve your fellow man.

Across nations, the spirit of God is awakening those most capable of light. These individuals are becoming God's elect of light. He is using them to arouse the truth and the light, according to the susceptibility of man, in order to manifest His glory on this planet. The elect, along with those capable of light, are guided to the community of light and wisdom, for only within this community does one learn to know God, nature, and man. This sacred community possesses the key to all mysteries, and the full knowledge of the inner workings of nature and creation. It is the primal depository of all power and truth entrusted from time immemorial.

As Universal Kabbalists, we are the depositories of a golden heritage of indescribable value, one that possesses the ancient secrets of the lost civilization of Atlantis. The time has come for us to disclose the spiritual wealth that grants freedom and immortality. Again, there can be no hope of higher happiness for humankind as long as we are bound by the corruptible, material essence that constitutes the main ingredient of our existence.

A final note: It is always good to know the truth, however one must be careful when speaking it. Heed the words of Jesus, who said, *Do not cast pearls before swine.* What he meant was that many are not prepared for the revelation of the truth. In order to receive the truth in the loving, enlightening spirit in which it is intended, one must have a strong nervous system and a good measure of wisdom. When you reveal the truth, the pearls, to people who do not possess these qualities, they attack. In other words, those who are not ready for the truth will react negatively in its presence. This is due to the fact that, in its directness, the truth is often painful. Take care when speaking the truth then, as uttering the truth before dark, evil people can bring you misfortune. Do not cast the truth on such individuals. Rather, as you treasure it within you, know that it will set you free, for Jesus also said, *Know the truth and the truth shall make you free.* Adorn yourself with the pearls of truth every day. Treasure them. Contemplate them. Then, lock them up in the secret chest that lies deep within you. This process will reinforce the truth in your own being, and you will radiate it outward. In turn, you will help others as they are indirectly supported by your inner truth and projected toward the light.

10

I AM THAT I AM

THE SECRET OF PRESENT-DAY human existence lies in the sentence: *I am*. Only beings that possess the external form we attribute to humans are able to think, feel, and imbue these words with will. Such physical form developed in a way that the frontward shape of the vaulted frontal lobe became the goal of all the forces working in the body. This vaulted frontal lobe and the *I Am* belong together. Early in the evolution of the human form, there was a stage when such a frontal lobe did not exist. At that time, the *I Am* could not be inwardly thought, willed, or felt. We must not misunderstand the sequence of events, however. The *I Am* was in existence even when the human body had not yet evolved. It could not, however, express itself in a form. Rather, it expressed itself in the world of the soul. In other words, the *I Am* predates the evolved human form we know today. Moreover, it is the very power of the *I Am* that, having united in the far-distant past with a human body lacking the present frontal lobe formation, impelled the forehead to assume its present shape. Hence it is that humans, by sinking deeply into the *I Am*, can feel the force that has molded them into their present form. This force is higher than the forces that are active within us today, in our ordinary lives.

I Am, also known as *I Am That I Am*, is a powerful spiritual formula that establishes a connection between the chanter and the Lord God; Holy Father, Almighty and Merciful One, Who has created all things, Who knows all things and can do all things, from Whom nothing is hidden, to Whom nothing is impossible. In other words, this is the entity from whom nothing can remain hidden, and to whom everything is possible. It is the One who allows you to penetrate the knowledge of hidden things, and understand their secret nature. Through *I Am*, we receive aid from the Most Holy *ADONAI*, whose Kingdom and Power shall have no end unto the Ages of the Ages. Amen.

I Am That I Am is also what Jesus meant when he said, *I and my Father are One*. It is the Holy Name of God, *Eheieh*. And the first name of God is Eheieh, the name of the divine essence, whose numeration is called Kether. Also referred to as the Macrosopus, Kether is the first sphere on the Tree of Life, and is also known as the crown. It is the first of the ten digits or spheres of the Tree of Life that represents the manifold expression of deity, conceived of as the creative power of the primal light. Kether signifies the simplest essence of divinity. It is the root of all things, a center of spiritual energy, full of ceaseless life, activity, and force. Standing for *Raysheeth ha gigoleem*, it is the first whirling, or impulse, and represents a concentration of light energy within the infinity of *Ain Soph* which sets in motion the process of being revealed. It is not, as yet, the will to create. Rather, it is the will to will. All beginnings, all seeds, all things represented by One, find their place in this, the sphere of the energy of *I Am That I Am*. Kether, then, is the door through which Ain Soph acts on the other Sephiroth. The will to create, known as Chokmah, is produced in this way. (For more information on Kether, Chokmah and the Spheres of the Tree of Life, refer to the book *Lifting the Veil*.)

The energy of Kether is the power to be conscious. The Archangel Metatron, the Angel of the presence, the prince of faces who, according to the ancient mythology was changed into a fiery flame, presides over Kether. It was through Metatron that the Lord spoke to Moses. And, in Kether you find the choir of angels known as the *Chayoth ha Qadesh*, or the holy living creatures. These are the four Kerubic beings seen by Ezekiel in his vision.

One is encouraged to read the opening of the book of Ezekiel. This records the prophet's vision of the Lord riding upon a fiery chariot of the Holy living creatures, accompanied by supernal vision and voices, as well as movements and upheaval on Earth. This revelation revealed an opening into the spiritual realms. It flung the door to the beyond wide open, so that the properly prepared individual, at the direct invitation of God, could mount the chariot as though it were a flaming Pegasus, and reach to the secret spiritual life that he labored for so long to reach.

The chariot of Ezekiel's vision (the Merkabah) was a 'mystic way' leading to the veritable heights of the Tree of Life, to the crown of all. It is the vehicle whereby the Kabbalist is carried directly to a face-to-face encounter with the highest divinity. The aim of all mystics, then, is to be a Merkabah rider. In this way, he might be enabled, while incarnated as a human being, to ascend to his spiritual paradise. Thus, the meaning of the chariot symbolism is enlightenment. As you can see, *I Am That I Am* or *Eheieh*, the first holy name of God from the Tree of Life is the root, source, and origin of all the other Divine Names, from whence they draw their life and virtue. It is the name Adam invoked in order to acquire knowledge of all created things. It contains the Power, Wisdom, and Virtue of the Spirit of God. The vast Mercy and Strength of God manifests in the life of those who work with it.

I Am is the revelation that Moses had in the burning bush: ...in the desert at the burning bush "the angel of the Lord appeared to Moses in a blazing fire from the midst of the bush, and identified Himself clearly.

"Moses said to God, "Suppose I go to the Israelites and say to them, 'The God of your fathers has sent me to you,' and they ask me, 'What is His Name?' Then what shall I tell them?"

"God said to Moses, 'I Am That I Am.' This is what you are to say to the Israelites: 'I Am has sent me to you.'"

"God also said to Moses, "Say to the Israelites, 'The Lord, the God of your fathers—the God of Abraham, the God of Isaac and the God of Jacob—has sent me to you.' This is my Name forever, the Name by which I am to be remembered from generation to generation." He is the eternal *I Am*.

The One who is speaking from the burning bush is the same, yesterday, today and forever. The angel of the Lord announces that He is Elohim, the self-existent One and beside Him there is none else. He is the Absolute I. He told Moses, "I Am That I Am." He is the same angel of the Lord who had appeared to Sarah, Hagar, Abraham and Isaac four hundred years earlier. Now He appears to Moses as the burning bush and reveals Himself as the "I Am That I Am."

While *I Am* looks like a simple formula, it conceals a mighty force that takes effect when made alive in the soul. As it connects you with the Holy Father, *I Am* connects you with your own spiritual force. This connection creates internal harmony and protection that extends to every aspect of your life. In order to work effectively with the mantra *I Am*, you must fill your entire inner being with its words by inhabiting their meaning with the full strength of your soul. Know that as you meditate on *I Am*, you become existence itself, without form, quality, past, present or future. In other words, this mantra relates the finite identity of the first *I am* with the infinite identity of the second *I am*. The first *I am*, then, is the personal reference. The second *I am* relates the I of self-identity to the Am of the existence of being.

It is essential for anyone who wants to follow the ways of the enlightened to work with the *I Am*. Think, *I Am* while simultaneously having the inner experience of something similar to: I rejoice that I, as an independent being, can participate in the work of healing and making the world a better place. Also experience something similar to: I will my own existence; I resolve to place myself in the whole context of the world. If you concentrate these experiences into a single, inner act of consciousness, while, at the same time, shift the whole force of your consciousness upwards into the region of the frontal lobe and the inner members of the brain beneath it, you will actually transfer yourself into a higher world. This is the world out of which your frontal lobe-formation has been brought into being.

A consistent, daily practice of listening to or chanting *I Am* from the Rootlight *Sounds of the Ether* CD will connect you to the higher world. You must display the patience to practice this meditation day by day, over and over again, for a long time. If you have this patience, then, after some time, you will notice a thought arising within you—no longer a mere concept but a thought thriving with life and force. Soon, this thought will reveal itself to you as if it were radiating light. Within this inner radiation of light, you will feel bountiful, blissful, happy and full of the joy of existence. A feeling will then permeate you. This feeling can only be described as joyful love in creative existence. A force imparts itself to the will as if the thought were radiating warmth through the will, energizing it. You can garner all of this by merging with the *I Am*. You will gradually realize that, by so sinking into the *I Am*, the highest intellectual, psychic, and moral powers are birthed in you.

I Am is a powerful way to reconnect with your true center, so that you may experience love, peace, and true joy in your life. Meditating on *I Am* with dedication, while chanting along with the track on the *Sounds of Ether* CD will initiate an integration of your mind, body, and spirit that enables you to unravel the mystery of your own being. In turn, you will come to unravel the understanding and nature of God. Indeed, as the mantra *I Am* becomes firmly fixed in the mind, all restrictive bonds and limitations are removed. Your sense of personal relatedness to the cosmic will be heightened, as you are connected with the healing energy of the universe, and showered with angelic gifts and blessings. This mantra is the essence of truth and the nature of reality. Chanting and/or listening to it will connect you with the higher world and surround you with the beneficial light of heaven. All you have to do is to chant along or listen to the *I Am* track on the *Sound of Ether* CD, and you will feel the heavenly connection on the spot, it works.

See page 159 for a suggested description to practice this meditation.

*I Am conceals a mighty force
that takes effect when made alive in the soul.*

*I Am connects you with your own spiritual force.
This connection creates internal harmony and
protection that extends to every aspect of your life.*

*I Am is a powerful way to reconnect with
your true center, so that you may experience love,
peace, and true joy in your life.*

11

CHILDREN

GOD, WHO CREATED ALL THINGS, in order that they may be submitted unto the will of Man, has included humankind in his project to bring his works to perfection by making Man participate in His Divine and Terrestrial work. Since the Fall of Adam and Eve, Man has a gross and terrestrial body, while his soul is spiritual and celestial. God has, in fact, made the whole earth and its inhabitants subject to him, and has given him means by which he may work with many spirits, which preside over manifold realms through God's bidding. Some of these celestial creatures govern the archangelic world, and others the angelic world. Some regulate the motion of the stars, some directly help humankind, and others continually sing the praises of God. There are also Saturnian, Jupiterian, Martian, Solar, Venusian, Mercurian and Lunarian spirits (all of whom correspond to the planets); there are also spirits of the elementals as well as of the heavens. They exist in fire, air, water, and others on earth, and will happily serve those who learn how to respect their nature and for whom they have affinity. Humankind has been allowed to profit from the good fortune and happiness that these divine spirits may impart, as long as he understands how to work with the invisible realm. Through the power of the word, you can cause the angels to help you, provided that you do not abuse this privilege by asking for negative outcomes. For cursed is the one who will use the name of God in vain, and who will employ for evil purposes the knowledge and good wherewith He has enriched us.

God has destined a guiding, protective spirit to each human being. This spirit is called a *genii*. The genii are elemental beings, such as ourselves, who are better able to render their services when we become aware of their presence and the rules that govern their existence. In other words, God has assigned a spirit, called a *genii*, to each human being, which watches over him and preserves him. Before age seven, our awareness of and connection to our *genii* is quite strong. Unfortunately, after age seven this link begins to fade. With the knowledge of the Divine Spiritual Wisdom contained in Universal Kabbalah along with the following *I Am I Am* meditation, you can help your child maintain his/her precious connection to their *genii*. With practice of such meditation, adults can progressively create the platform whereby their connection can be restored. Enabling children to keep this heavenly connection is beneficial in that it can help guide them safely through this complex world.

Time and space have changed. The world is changing, and we are changing. Clairvoyant children are being born in large numbers with the impetus to strive toward a new kind of group consciousness that can no longer be suppressed. Therefore, it is important that we recognize our children as the brave and fearless guardians of the future. Parents and teachers must work with and for children so that they are properly protected, nurtured, molded, and guided. One tool that parents, in particular, can give to their children is to help them maintain their connection to the guiding, protective spirit each of us receives at birth. In addition, we must remember that children are highly susceptible to adult influence. It is our responsibility to set them on the path toward positive and productive living, so that they evolve into ideal citizens of the universe. This is best achieved when we lead by example. When we live in accordance with high ideals, while demonstrating the principles of good physical and mental health, we become the living models of that which we wish our children to be and become. To do anything less is to be a hypocrite.

Mental balance is the key to a child's success in both playtime and learning. Indeed, a child's level of social and academic accomplishment is directly related to his or her level of mental and emotional health. Eventually, of course, this translates into other forms of success later on in life. Therefore, it is incumbent upon us to foster each child's innate, individual gifts without encumbering him or her with our particular desires. We must resist the urge to live vicariously through our children by making them into the image of ourselves. Rather, we must allow them to be who they are. A child with an aptitude for the arts should not be forced to be a doctor or scientist. Help your children to recognize their special talents and qualities. Watch and analyze their tendencies and inclinations, and encourage them to choose a path that fits their interests. Above all, allow your children to grow up with their original purity, spontaneity, and creativity intact.

Through teaching our children meditations along with the *I Am I Am* mantra, we become the spiritual guardians who show them a higher and simpler way of life. This is an excellent meditation to do with your child in order to improve his or her physical and mental well-being. Indeed, doing this meditation for as little as three minutes can help give a child of any age the confidence and security that is so important and necessary in this life. You can meditate along with the child using the "I Am" track on the *Sounds of the Ether* CD. It is not only important for adults to be in touch with their heart, but also, our children will especially benefit if we encourage them with meditations such as the following, to connect with their protective guiding spirit. Please note that what is described in the following exercises is appropriate for people of all ages.

CONNECTING WITH YOUR GUIDING SPIRIT
The following *I Am I Am* Meditation is designed to help you draw from the infinite source of power and strength within. It will open the doors of your heart and let the power of the Spirit flow in and through you. By opening the heart, we gain access to our Holy Guardian Angel, characterized by a strong manifestation of intuition. This is the final resting place for the shaktic power after its ascent, and it is the ideal to which mystics aspire. Therefore, meditations such as this one, are designed to prepare our minds, bodies, and consciousness for the liberation of the Divine and Sweet Fire buried deep inside us. By chanting the sacred mantra, *I Am That I Am* you are vibrating the very name of the Lord, God of Abraham, God of Isaac, and God of Jacob, that He revealed to

Moses. After the revelation, God then said, "This is my Name forever, and thus I am to be remembered throughout all generations." Therefore, when you chant *I Am I Am*—the name of God—God will start flowing through you, for the power of the name of God is such that whosoever pronounces it with the tongue will purify his or her entire being. As a result, the purified being becomes God, forever.

Chanting this mantra, then, connects you with Moses' experience in the burning bush. It links you to the Divine Flame of Fire, which burst forth from the Holy ground on the Mountain of God. Moreover, chanting mantras such as *I Am That I Am* while maintaining a simultaneous mental connection with the Sun awakens powers heretofore unknown, and re-awakens those that are dormant by evoking the inner spiritual force, manifested as the Holy Flame of Divine Fire. We chant *I Am That I Am* to pierce to the core of truth and understand the nature of reality. *I Am That I Am* expresses the very origin of God. It will cause that immeasurable force of high spiritual vibration to infuse your being, while moving and shifting your life to the highest moral goal and self perfection.

The following meditation connects you with that imponderable Divine fire from within that directs the ever increasing urge of your inner self towards merging with the most sacred temple of all, for harmony and balance.

Meditation: I Am, I Am

POSITION:
Sit with a straight spine. Place your right hand on your knee in wisdom pose, (thumb and forefinger pressed together). Your left hand should be at the level of your heart, pointing towards the right with the palm flat and fingers straight. Your eyes should remain mostly closed and focused on your left hand. As you begin, you want to keep your left hand six inches away from your chest. As you say the first *I Am*, however, you will want to move it about six inches closer. As you say the second *I Am*, the hand will then move back to the starting position. Keep repeating the sequence.

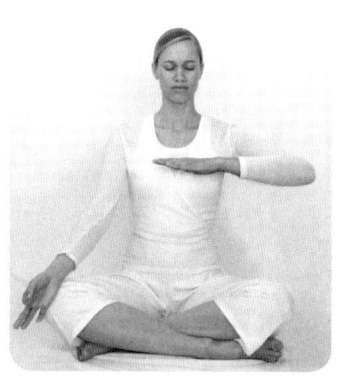

TIME:
Start with a few minutes each day, adding more as you progress and eventually working up to 11 minutes.

COMMENTS:
Your chest is a great ocean of energy. When you chant *I Am*, feel it in the depth of your soul. Do it slowly and put your self into it. The closer I AM means, *I AM who I know myself to be*, while the farther I AM means, *I AM that which is greater than I know myself to be*. As you do the meditation, feel light energy enter your chest and heart, surrounding you with a field of bright light that takes your mind into an expansive peacefulness. With each *I Am*, feel the sun of healing, brilliant light rising in your heart and your entire body be filled with its illuminating radiance. Let all the worries of the day drop away as you circulate the sacred sound, *I Am I Am*. You are listening to the eternal ocean through it.

In addition to meditations, various mudras can be used to develop different aptitudes. Having a child touch the thumb to the middle finger develops discipline. Having the thumb touch the ring finger heightens nervous strength. Having the thumb touch the pinkie finger heightens communicative abilities.

Also, teaching your child the beautiful *Prayer of Love, Peace, and Light (page 172)* can be extremely beneficial. It has an harmonizing effect upon the emotional state and counteracts harmful energies. In other words, it keeps unwanted influences away and attracts heavenly blessings. They can recite it in the morning upon arising and/or at night before they go to sleep.

In addition, as soon as an adult or child recites *Triple Mantra* the heavens have to automatically take over for their protection. *Triple Mantra* moves the heavens and invokes the luminous beings to protect you. If you or your child feels endangered or stuck, recite or work with the Rootlight *Triple Mantra* CD. It works. These special tools can help children face this complex world safely and gracefully.

TRIPLE MANTRA:
Ad Guray Nameh
Jugad Guray Nameh
Sat Guray Nameh
Siri Guru Devay Nameh
Ad Such
Jugad Such
HehBEE Such
Nanaka O See BEE Such
Ad Such
Jugad Such
HehBEH Such
Nanaka O See BEH Such

Two voices exist within each of us. They are the voice of the ego, which is closely aligned with the head, and the voice of the soul, which is closely aligned with the heart. Those who follow the head lose their way to the path of truth and clarity. Those who follow the heart, however, are granted the mental peace and calm that allows the path of truth to automatically stretch out before them. It is imperative, then, that we work to serve the soul rather than the ego. Direct all your passions to the service of God. This, and this alone, will make you happy and healthy.

The time for thinking someone else can heal you is over. Now, more than ever, each of us must take responsibility for our own physical wellness and spiritual evolution. In other words, we must take responsibility for our own healing and transformation. In this regard, the book *The Divine Doctor* is a major treatise on the art of self-healing and the secret of a permanent cure. By working with it you will create a platform for self healing. There is also the Harmonyum Healing system, which activates the original seed and awakens the threefold soul, born of the threefold spirit, from the threefold body into self consciousness and self knowledge. It is extremely beneficial for adults and children. Harmonyum brightens your energy, wipes out karma, and increases your sense of personal relatedness to the infinite identity. Above all seek and find your direct link with the Lord, and consciously maintain it regardless of what is going on around you. This link with the Divine is the source of all power and goodness that creates miracles. Indeed, miracles manifest when we attune ourselves to the power of "I Am I Am" within. For, in reality, we are nothing on our own. But with God, all things can be accomplished. Humility is an essential component to finding your link with the Divine, and the most humble on this earth are the most high in the house of God. The above meditation is a spiritual cure that enables both you and your child to get in touch with the voice of the soul. In so doing, it acts as a centering force, putting you in the right places and helping you prepare for the difficult times ahead.

The sacred wisdom contained in Universal Kabbalah demonstrates the effectiveness of the Word, while helping you to understand the application and implication of time proven truths. The average man will not understand the depth and effectiveness of working with the Word. He will not understand that working with the Word allows you to gracefully face the challenges of time and space. The Word, however, is the greatest power available to man. As you absorb this Divine Spiritual Wisdom, your consciousness expands, and you are filled with so much light that you become unshakable. You receive a whole host of benefits, as well as the guidance and help you need to experience a happy, successful, and fulfilling life.

Therefore, work with the Divine Spiritual Wisdom so that you can gain the experience of your own strength, your own purity, and your own infinity. Allow our sacred wisdom to make your life one of indescribable joy. Understand that as you apply the sacred wisdom, your mind and heart are synchronized in praise of the Lord. You are touched by His vastness, and, in turn, your mind is cleansed of negativity. As a result, you can see the light of your own soul, and from the light of the soul you see that which is bountiful and beautiful. This is nothing less than an act of love. By lifting the veil that blankets your soul, our sacred teachings give you a clearer vision of your life's purpose, your reason for being here.

The Divine Spiritual Wisdom contained in Universal Kabbalah causes the channel of Beatitude to open itself in its sublimity. It creates within Man, the spiritual wedding or that which is known as *Mysterium Conjunctionis of the Alchemists*. As a result, man, who is lost in the ocean of Being without boundaries and place, is transported up to the confines of Omneity. Thus, you realize the greater presence and power that is God, and you are reminded of where you came from, of why you are here, of where you will return to, of your true destiny, including the infinite and loving omnipresence and might of our creator. Thus one becomes a pure channel of love, peace, and light to all. Then, grace and blessings keep flowing into the life of Man whose nature has been transformed in a sweet and incomprehensible merger with the Will and Mercy of the Lord. In other words, this beautiful and sacred wisdom, through the mystical marriage of the lamb causes spirit to spiritualize matter and turns a human into pure spiritual Gold.

12

THE WAY OF THE HEART

YOGA FEVER IS SPREADING, and many are now practicing some form of yoga. Although the more physically based forms of yoga are beneficial, they are not enough to usher you into the spiritual worlds. In order to enter the spiritual worlds, you need to open your heart center. No amount of physical exercise can help you accomplish this task, because spirituality is not a quality of the physical body. Indeed, man is in possession of both a physical body and a spiritual body, therefore he is dual in nature. Keep in mind, that which is physical is physical, and that which is spiritual is spiritual. Material things only affect their own kind. Therefore, physical means, such as eating or abstaining from a certain food and/or working out, do not provide the necessary condition for spiritual consciousness. In other words, there is no exercise regime or diet that assures spiritual unfolding and development. Daily exercise tunes our physical body, not our spiritual body, and food itself does not have any direct affect on our spiritual nature. If performing a series of physical exercises were enough, then the 84 yogic asanas would lengthen your life, but you can do them for years and then die without ever meeting God. You need to open your heart in order to meet God; for God is not in your head, He is in your heart.

Having said that, one should strive to keep the body in good health, thereby making it a temple worthy of the spirituality which manifests from within. To be sure, a well-balanced diet, in combination with moderate physical exercise, contributes to the overall health, welfare, and harmony of both mind and body, thus making increased spiritual development more possible. Extremism with regard to eating is detrimental. Suppressing our desire for food and need for exercise, and/or allowing the body to degrade due to a lack of proper nutrition or long fasts is a mistake. An ill body can prevent the spiritual property from having the proper kind of medium for expression. If we were to eliminate the physical and material things of life, there would be no purpose left for the existence of spiritual knowledge and power.

As previously stated, the opening of the heart is a purely spiritual matter. To be perfectly clear, the spirit does not dwell in the familiar physical body. That body is composed of frail matter, and is the cause of our depravity and our mortality. Rather, the spirit dwells in the invisible spiritual body we inhabit, that is the temple of God in us. This body is fundamentally organized from a transcendental, metaphysical, and invisible substance that is both incorruptible and immortal. Moreover, it is complete with invisible spiritual organs and senses that correspond to physical counterparts. Just as the physical body has various organs and senses that enable it to perform complicated work and allow us to be conscious of physical things, so too our spiritual body has various organs and senses that allow us to perceive spiritual worlds, things, and beings. Now, things only work in their proper environment. The spiritual realms are perfectly suited to spiritual beings and the spiritual nature of man, but not to physical man. Absolute truth does not exist for the sensuous man; it exists only for the interior and spiritual man who possesses suitable interior organs capable of receiving the absolute truth of the transcendental worlds. These organs constitute a spiritual faculty which cognizes spiritual objects as objectively and naturally as the exterior senses perceive external, physical phenomena. In order to see the unseen, we need spiritual eyes. In order to hear the unheard, we need spiritual ears. In order to know the unknown, we need intuitive intelligence. Unfortunately, the interior faculty of spiritual man, that sensorial function necessary for the perception of the metaphysical worlds, is not yet known to those who only cognize on the external realm, for it is a mystery of the Kingdom of God. As long as the temple of God in man, the heart center, remains closed, the spiritual body of man with its spiritual interior organs remains inactive. The opening of the heart center and the spiritual body is the noblest goal of all spiritual practices whose ultimate goal is to unite Man with God in Spirit and Truth.

Interestingly, the actions of our spiritual body are not related to our bodily animal functions at the same time that the spiritual body exists independently of corporeal life. The faculties of the material body are corporeal and, therefore, do not have the power of immortality. Their action is non-existent once the spiritual body departs at death. Indeed, the indestructible form of spiritual man was created by the will of the creator without any physical working of matter. When the bonds that link the spiritual body with the physical body are destroyed, the corpse is left to disintegrate. As the material body dissolves and is reduced to inanimate ashes lacking in action or virtue, it returns all that it has received from the Earth back to the Earth. The spiritual body, now freed from the shackles of matter with which it has never been directly united, goes toward the lower or higher astral planes according to the extent to which you have become purified. The purification that leads to the higher astral plane is reached through service and the path of the heart. The lower astral plane is reached when we have been corrupted by the three lower centers.

How does one initiate an opening of his/her heart center? The opening of the heart center is initiated by living in accordance with the precepts of the Way of the Heart. To follow the Way of the Heart is to live a life characterized by kindness, compassion, charity, humanness, forgiveness, benevolence, understanding, and service. All other methods are merely substitutes. Reading all manner of spiritual books and/or going to yoga every day does not change one's interior perception and state of consciousness. These practices do not open the heart. It is the practice of chanting mantra, working with the Sun, obeying the Laws of Nature, and following the Way of the Heart that opens the heart by effecting the Transmutation, or what is know to the Rose Croix Kabbalists as the *Magnum Opus*.

Evolved beings follow the Way of the Heart. The most tender and sensitive towards mankind, such beings are always ready to share another's trouble, sorrow, depression, or despair. They are prepared to use their words to console any and every person. They are willing to offer their service, and provide sympathy to those in need. They do not shrink away from personal sacrifices of time, money, pleasure, or comfort. We must adopt the ways of the evolved and cultivate sympathy for our fellowman, learning to share in his troubles and his despair. This is the joy of life, and whoever truly experiences it will find that it becomes so great that the heart and soul are filled. For such individuals, it matters not if they receive less in the way of material comforts or prestige than their fellows, because the light of their kindness, sympathy, ever-growing love, and virtuous heart fill the soul with light. They want for nothing in life, and lack nothing in life, for they have become the kings of life. These are the true healers, the true servants of the universe, and the possessors of the true wine that can unpretentiously and unassumingly heal others with a glance, a kind word, a simple touch, and the presence of their nature. Indeed, real healing is affected when one is in sympathy with another's trouble and lends a helping hand. He who can send from his eye the glance of love that proves the divine sympathy and help he is anxious to give, bears the true mark of healing power.

Something must be said about the method of physical purification dear to the hearts of the light agents of the intellectual plane: vegetarianism. This timeless practice does lessen a person's willingness to focus his/her attention only on the physical plane. However, physical self-purification means little if we do not simultaneously purge the mental and emotional bodies of such destructive patterns as negativity, spiteful speech, destructive emotions, and other inner qualities that are a hundredfold more harmful than the karma acquired from eating meat. A person who is a mental and emotional vegetarian works in the realm of the heart, for he/she thinks and feels with compassion and understanding for fellow human beings. To be a true vegetarian is to think right, feel right, speak right, act right, behave right and eat right. When we cleanse our lives of harmful thoughts, emotions, speech, deeds and eating habits, then we are practicing mental, astral and physical vegetarianism.

As we have discussed, man is dual in nature. While the heart is the seat of the Christic light, the love nature, and the love of all that is good and wholesome, it is also the seat of malice, envy, jealousy, anger, and evil thoughts. The true purpose of life is to open your heart, purging it of negative influences so that you become a channel of God. You are not here to glorify your little self, for a candle that burns alone serves only itself and its light slowly diminishes. The burning candle that lights the path for others, on the other hand, serves and uplifts the whole of humanity. Its light becomes brighter and brighter. Therefore, the true idea of life is to serve and uplift others from the power of your Heart. You cannot truly practice effective spiritual work before your heart center has been opened and regenerated by its positive powers. Once a true opening of the heart has occurred, the faculties of precognition are awakened, becoming useful tools for communicating with the divine spiritual beings during prayer.

In order to rise above the endless modifications of your fundamental animal instincts, you must open your heart center correctly. For the highest degree of human culture, which the world has until now maintained, has still not brought us any further along the path of evolution than to cover over this fundamental instinct of animal man with a fine coating. There can be no hope of higher happiness for mankind as long as the corruptible, material essence, expressed through the lower chakras, constitutes the main ingredient of existence. You must open your heart in order to make the mortal immortal, and the corruptible incorruptible.

Christ spoke about the mysteries of regeneration with his most intimate friend while he was still on this earth. The opening of the heart brings regeneration. Regeneration is a loosening and detachment of this impure and corruptible matter which keeps our immortal being chained in bonds, and the life of the repressed, active spiritual power sunk, as it were, in the sleep of death. Working with the heart is the means by which one removes this ferment and transforms death and misery in us in order to again set free our original, suppressed power. The heart, then, is the true medicine for mankind revealed by the spirit of God. It is the table of the Lord laid for everyone, where the true bread of the angels is prepared. When you have raised yourself and purified your consciousness, you become imbued with new life, and you are automatically drawn upward. Reintegration is therefore an effect, not a cause.

The opening of the heart unites us to the spiritual world. As a result we are enlightened through wisdom, guided by truth, and nourished by the flames of love. Unknown powers unfold in us in order to overcome the darkness. Our whole being is renewed, and we are empowered to become an actual, dwelling God. We are granted the power to oversee nature and intercourse with the higher worlds, as well as the visible enjoyment of intercourse with God. The blindfold of ignorance falls from our eyes, the chains of illusion are broken, and we have the freedom of God's children. The universe is one symphony and each person is one note. Happiness lies in becoming perfectly attuned to the harmony of the universe.

The essence of life and leadership lies in the Way of the Heart and in the conquering of the negative karmic influences that create duality in your life. The Great Work is performed by restoring your in faculties the same law, the same order, and the same regularity by which all beings are directed in Nature. True divine spiritual work is done by acting no longer in our own name, but in that of the living God. Utilize the Divine Spiritual Wisdom, gifted to us, to open your heart and confront your negative karmic influences, so that you may move to a state of divinity. During these eight years, as the darkness of the world grows denser, increase the power and strength of your inner light through mantra and prayer so that you are able to overcome the world and become a demonstration of the eternal life and light. Do not allow negativity to dim your light. Let it blaze forth within you.

More than ever, the Divine Spiritual Wisdom that we teach is becoming the leading light of the Age of Aquarius, or the Age of the Heart. It reveals the sacred blueprint by which we must live in this age in order to experience the grace and divinity of universal intelligence. These teachings are designed to make your journey through and beyond this transition happy, successful, and fulfilling. This work contains a real science; it is founded on pure and genuine truth. It is the promised inheritance of the elect who are capable of light. The practice of this sacred wisdom is the fulfillment of the divine union with the children of men.

The deep mysteries that we teach, passed down from the lineage of the Community of Light, will be of interest to those people who are desirous of nurturing the highest form of light and love, and manifesting that on earth. Many are called to this heavenly science, but only those who have sufficiently advanced, gratefully and humbly understanding the sacred nature of the teachings shared, along with a desire to use these teachings in service, will remain. As you commit to and learn this Divine Spiritual Wisdom you will become a beacon of light and love, an instrument of peace in the world, and you will join the lineage of the Community of Light as a true servant of God. To be sure, we are the Apostles of this Fountain of Light, and our work is unlike any other. Our sacred teachings not only show the way to illumination, but they hold the Sun of Light and the wisdom that leads to it. Let mantra be your working tool. Practice with the Word, and you will have a daily living communion with the Fountain of Light, the Logos or Word. The practice of chanting mantras will not only connect you with the higher worlds, it will initiate the personal change and growth that spreads positive change throughout the world. When you consistently use mantras, you become a healing vehicle whereby the Earth is revitalized. Indeed, the effectiveness of the words of power we use, when spread, could change the entire world. With the healing vibration of mantras embedded in the earth, we can all return to a state of perfect harmony.

As you practice this heavenly wisdom, you will find the confirmation of the righteousness of the spiritual truths within yourself, and you will see the potency and visible results produced by the mantras we recommend. Each day, as you perform your spiritual practice, face east towards the rising sun, which is symbolic of the Fountain of Light. The period of sunrise is an especially excellent time to connect with the healing forces of the universe in order to ask for healing and gain spiritual attunement. During the beneficial waxing moon, devote a portion of each day to aligning yourself with the potent healing and constructive powers of nature. Working with the Word will increase your sense of personal connection to the cosmic, and shower you with heavenly light, gifts, and blessings. It harmonizes you with the healing energy of the universe. Use the ritual outlined on page 171 to call upon the creative strength and vitality of the spiritual centers so that you can heal yourself, your loved ones and, indeed, the world. The doors of heaven will open, and its blessings will begin to flow toward you. Recite daily some of the mantras on the Rootlight Sacred Music Series. They will open your heart, illumine you, align you with the Divine, and protect you.

Your chest is a great ocean of energy. In it you find the heart. The peace for which every soul strives, and which is the true nature of God and the utmost goal of man, is found in the heart or by following the heart. The source of every truth is hidden in every human's heart. The heart is the seat of life, and life is the outcome of harmony. The whole secret of creation is harmony. The harmony of the universe is life itself. And it is life that every one desires. It is life that is the real source of healing. The temple of God resides in the heart. It is the essence of all beings, the progressive, higher self within the self. Always throbbing, always beating, the heart is the ultimate chanter, and the beat of the heart is the rhythm of your soul. The heart chants continuously, relating to the presence of God—the Creative force that continues, uninterrupted. This relationship is perfectly balanced and harmonious. Whether or not you pay attention to it, the heart beats on. The beauty herein is that the moment your heart stops beating, you are released from this world of illusion called Maya. Unfortunately, humankind has replaced the precious internal temple of the heart with the external form of worship. This is a grave error. We must not lose the temple that is the heart. Practicing these types of exercises enables you to align your mental, astral, and physical bodies, so that you can become aware of the true, initial cause of imbalance and illness. This, in turn, will provide you with an opportunity to empower and heal yourself by seeking out those situations and persons in your life that need to be addressed and tended to in order to reach a healing point of resolution.

The first part of this "I Am" Meditation is an empowering, healing exercise designed to cleanse the lymph glands and the lungs in the upper chest and helps prevent breast cancer and heart attack. It also helps balance the right and left hemispheres of the brain because the hands are the servants of the brain. The benefits of this meditation are both physical and metaphysical. Incorporate the "I Am" exercise and meditation into your daily spiritual practice. It is an excellent addition. Recite this sacred sound as you face East towards the rising Sun that is symbolic of the Fountain of Light. This can be done for 40 days. It will connect you with your heart, illumine your soul, and align you with the Divine.

Meditation to Connect with Your Heart

STEP I: WARM-UP *(3 minutes)*
Sit as calmly as you can, in any posture that does not cause pain. Relax the arms at the sides with the palms facing upward. As rapidly as possible, alternately bend the elbows so that the forearms come up toward the heart center. Do not bend the wrists or hands, and do not touch the chest. As you proceed with this rapid fanning movement, the arms will begin to feel as if they are moving automatically. Try to maintain a balance in the rhythmic motion of your hands. If your hands hit each other, it means that this balance has been upset. After a couple of minutes you may feel sweat on your forehead. Do this first part for at least three minutes.

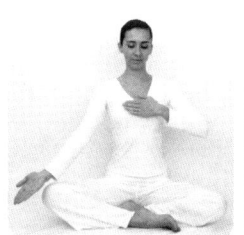

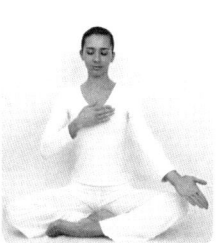

STEP II. CONNECT WITH YOUR HEART *(11 minutes)*
Put your hands on your heart, listen to your heart beat and feel like you are at home. You are resting in the center of your self. Chant along with "I Am I Am" on the *Sounds of the Ether* CD. As you chant *I Am*, feel it in the depth of your soul. Connect with this Divine flame of light that burns within yourself, and let it shine forth and welcome all that is good, all that is healing, all that will aid humankind and its growth in this world. Connect with your heart so that this Divine candlelight may burn brightly, holding your mind, body and spirit, so that these things of goodness and love may come to you, and God in all his wisdom may guide you towards those healing paths that you are meant to walk.

(continued on next page)

Step III: Send Love, Peace, and Light to the World

Love before me
Love behind me
Love at my left
Love at my right
Love above me
Love below me
Love in me
Love in my surroundings
Love to all
Love to the universe

Peace before me
Peace behind me
Peace at my left
Peace at my right
Peace above me
Peace below me
Peace in me
Peace in my surroundings
Peace to all
Peace to the universe

Light before me
Light behind me
Light at my left
Light at my right
Light above me
Light below me
Light in me
Light in my surroundings
Light to all
Light to the universe

13

THE HEART CENTER

The Sun, Moon, and Earth dance within us. Life is the art of keeping this dance in balance. Such balance is beautifully achieved through the heart. The heart is the source of manifestation and the medium between man and God. An open heart keeps darkness at bay, and there is no power more exalted than that of the power of prayer through an open heart. The heart is ruled by the Sun as a planetary body, and the hands are its working organs. On the Tree of Life the heart, which corresponds to the sphere Tiphareth, is a projection of Kether, the Crown. The Divine Name attributed to Kether is the name of the Father: Eheieh, I Am, The Most Holy Ancient One. Its projection is Beauty or Mildness, represented by the Divine Name *Eloah Va-Daath*, and the angelic names, Shinanim, Melakim, kings. Thus, by the union of Justice and Mercy we obtain beauty or clemency, and the second trinity of the Sephiroth is complete. This Sephirah, with sometimes the fourth, fifth, seventh, eighth, and ninth Sephiroth, are spoken of as ZOIR ANPIN or *Zauir Anpin*, the Lesser Countenance, or Microprosopus. The six Sephiroth, of which Zauir Anpin is composed, are then called His six members. He is also called *Melekh*, the King.

Tiphareth is the highest manifestation of ethical life, and the sum of all goodness. It relates to the Hindu Hari, the other name for Shri Krishna, because as a divine incarnation he was one in whom both spirit and matter were in complete equilibrium. The heart center, or fourth chakra, is the home of the conscious principle and the seat of prana, which is life.

From birth to death, prana plays a crucial role. At birth, it is the air that gives energy during delivery. At death, it collects all vital energy from the body and flows out, leaving a lifeless corpse behind. During life, prana resides in the area from the nostrils to the lungs. Situated in the cavity of the mouth, prana allows food to pass through to the stomach, while its location near the heart preserves life from destruction. Prana further acts to regulate the other elements of the body, effectively keeping them in balance. With the help of prana, we are able to move, see, think, and hear. A shift in our attitudes affects the speed and rhythmic cycle of the prana in our bodies. Thus, the heart center is governed by the element of air, known as Prana Vayu, and it dwells in the chest region. It is the air that we breathe, and it is rich in life giving negative ions. Air is not only tactile; it is the protective element in the body. It is the vital force that keeps the organs healthy and the blood circulating. Again, the fourth chakra rules the chest region, known as vayu-granthi, including the five principle glands: the lungs, heart, thymus, cell producers, and all their subsidiaries. When you are in possession of strong vayu-granthi, self-control, balanced temperament, purity of thought, and unselfishness are yours.

The fourth chakra, located at the heart, relates to healing and compassion. This chakra, the heart center, is the central chakra in which the individual becomes aware of the behavioral patterns of his life. It acts both as the balancing point between the three lower chakras and the three higher chakras, and is simultaneously influenced by them. From the fourth chakra, energy flows both downward and upward. Female and male energies merge. Therefore, it is vital to balance the energies of the heart. When you do so, the desires of the lower triangle are calmed and your attention is turned toward the pursuit of higher aims. The emotional self evolves and the cosmic mind is accessed. A flow of energy begins to move upward from the heart, inspiring the individual to transcend the intellectual understanding of divinity that characterizes the third chakra, and move into a direct experience of the divine within himself. In this way, the heart brings you grace and grace takes away temptation, anger, lust, greed, and unvirtuous and unrighteous living. By living through the heart, you relate to your spirit and flow of the soul, and you feel the total divinity within. With a heart pure in spirit, you are able to perceive divine grace in all things. Indeed, heart-centered living is a manifestation of divinity. Again, this connection to the divine surpasses mere intellectual understanding and infuses the individual with the oneness of life through the heart. Such an individual is vibrating from the heart region, the seat of the celestial wishing tree.

The heart center, or fourth chakra, then, is one of the two centers which are in direct contact with the higher self, and through which soul energy and the other higher energy enter our being. (The second entrance is the head center, in almost the exact center of the head in the vicinity of the pineal gland.) The heart center is also called the plane of the cosmic mind based on this unity with the absolute. It is the dwelling place of the emotional self. This is due to the fact that the thymus gland is located in the heart region. This gland is responsible for the flow of electrical impulse in the body. Sense perception is electrical in nature. Each change in our emotional patterns is registered by the heart and, in turn, regulates the body chemistry that is understood by the mind to be a certain feeling.

The heart is far more than a machine that pumps pure blood into the body and conveys waste-charged blood back to the lungs. It is also a center of feelings, a psychic center. The heart center is also the source of all transpersonal psychic phenomena. Initiates emphasize the importance of opening this chakra through love, transforming the personal into the impersonal, and filling one's life with poetry. Poetry itself is full of heart in all its vibrations. When one vibrates exclusively in the three lower chakras, it is very difficult to develop a positive attitude. However, vibrating from the heart center causes a person to develop good healthy habits, by attuning his own vibratory rate with that of the cosmos. Working with the heart and breath allows one simultaneous control over the breath patterns and the heart, creating positive vibratory frequencies. A good attitude in turn helps develop the heart center, while each wrong breath is an injury to the organism. Furthermore, we increase our positive attitudes by working closely with the cycle of the planets and the laws of the universe. You can overcome all the challenges of time and space so easily by faith in the God of your heart and living from your true self. Therefore, when caught in the trap of time, remember that you can be saved as well as pleased by the God of your heart.

Deep within you lies the eternal flow of life, and the strength, pure truth, and light of God. Through the practice of Naam, we can learn to direct the life force to the heart, where we can receive the baptism of Spiritual Fire. Naam is the heavenly food of the most perfect and God-like beings, a heavenly diet that gives us radiant health and a path to fulfilling our destiny. Naam is the higher and superior form of spiritual food for the advanced human race. Open your heart and vibrate the Word, and your inner being will be deeply imbued with the heavenly, protective color of the Love and Light of the Creator. You will be showered with His Mercy, and His eternal Goodness will lead you. His boundless Charity will inflame you, and His supreme Divinity will direct you. Open your heart and vibrate the Word, and you will find the gate of salvation. Work with the Naam, and Naam will carry you across the poisonous ocean of worldly challenges with grace, and cause the God of incomparable beauty who fulfills our hopes and aspirations to sit in your heart. Vibrate the Naam and your tongue will be imbued with the Lord's Essence. Vibrate the Naam and your ten trillion cells will by imbued with the Love of the Lord. Those whose hearts are not filled with the Lord's Name will see all their affairs become worthless and empty. Those who have not yet opened their heart and developed the lost inner faculty that allows them to perceive the hidden, eternal truths, will feel depressed, empty, lonely, and/or restless. Therefore, vibrate and drink in the sublime essence of the Naam, so that the Divinity of God may bless you, His piety warm you, and His love preserve you. *The Seal of Higher Destiny* delivers the cooling, soothing water of the Naam, thereby neutralizing the burning fire of bad karma.

The Glory of those who open their hearts to the Creator and serve others is manifest throughout the world. You will find truth in your heart. The essence of Naam is the practice of Truth. The crown of the sacred wisdom is bestowed upon those who vibrate the Naam; they are forever blessed by heaven. Vibrate the Naam and the radiant mark of purity will be written on your forehead. Vibrate the Naam, and the dormant power that makes one all-knowing, peaceful, and full of light will be gracefully and sweetly aroused. When we vibrate the Naam, we expand the breath and contract through the heart, which causes us to digest heavenly light. The Creator is pleased with those who vibrate the Naam that enshrines their minds and hearts with the Sublime Essence of the Name of the Lord. Liberate yourself by tuning into the power of Naam to open your heart. Naam will create a connection between you and the higher world. This form of communion is like a sweet, spiritual wine; it is a communion of the soul with the realms of light.

Meditation to Brighten Your Radiance

Position:
Sit in easy pose, spine straight. Place the two hands about 12 inches to either side of the ears, palms facing forward, fingers pointing straight up towards the ceiling. The elbows are not pressed into the sides, but are held away from the body a bit. Bend the index finger down and curl it under the thumb (Gyan Mudra). The rest of the fingers are held side by side, pointing straight up. Hold the position steady.

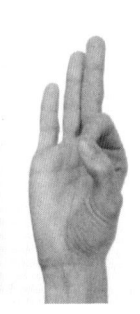

Focus the eyes on the tip of the nose

Breath:
Make your lips into a very clear "O," and breathe long and deep through the "O" mouth.

Music:
Ad Such (Track 2, *Sounds of the Ether,* or Track 3, *Green House*)

Time:
Continue for 11 minutes. To end, inhale deeply through the nose, hold the breath, come into a state of shunnia (zero) and synchronize your entire being. Hold 20 seconds. Relax.

Comments:
"In life we must increase our spiritual wisdom and experience so that we may live life gracefully with higher consciousness. The goal of this Divine Spiritual Wisdom is to allow one to live life with the maximum light and effectiveness and also with humility. You shall project out by your radiance. You shall be loved and honored by your excellence, or stupidity, as the case may be. As a human being you must always remember that you are a beam of light. That's your identity."

14

THE WAY OF SERVICE

ONE LAW OF NATURE HOLDS that if someone comes to you in need of help, and you do all that you can for that person, you will be rewarded within seven days. Each and every person that comes to you in need, then, is an opportunity to enhance your personal happiness. Indeed, they are blessings in your life; for your happiness and pain in the present and/or future are directly related to how many come to you, and how many you serve or deny. The more people you serve, the more people God sends you. If you serve others, God will serve you, for if you can hold another who is falling apart in the flow of spirit, if you can bring them to the Divine Spiritual Wisdom, you have attained a state of consciousness that is the virtue of all virtues. If, however, you give up on somebody who could have been rescued, who could have been saved, who could have been delivered to the house of God, you have committed a sin. Give God the chance to make you happy by striving to make others happy. When you truly understand that those who come to you in need are representative of the opportunity for God to bless you, you will not turn away. Above all, just remember that all you need to do is touch one heart and you will create a ripple of love, peace, and light that extends beyond the radius of that initial interaction.

It doesn't matter how much you study, how much you read, how much you know, and how powerful you think you are, you shall never have the grace to penetrate the heart of God, if you do not serve others and venerate the Word that is God. Your word shall never have the power to make the universe serve you, because you have not served others and understood that the Word is God. Service brings humility, and humility leads to the perfection of love. The mysteries of God are revealed to the humble. Humility is the throne of love; unless this throne is firmly established, love is ignored. Christ is a symbol of love and humility. And God is love. Serving allows you to love the God within an individual. The moment that happens, you become an universal soul. Love is the experience of sacrifice within oneself. Let an enemy come before you, and totally melt the coldness of his heart away with the flood of love, and service. Therefore, we invite you to learn the Divine Spiritual Wisdom contained in Universal Kabbalah, so that you may grow spiritually, glow like the bright Sun, and serve by being a lighthouse. Serve by being the answer and not the question. Serve by removing the obstacles present in the lives of others. When you serve in such a way, God removes the obstacles from your life.

Learn our sacred teachings, work with the Word, and try to know the unknown, and everybody in the human world, in the animal kingdom, in the mineral kingdom, and in the angelic world will know you. Serve others and God will hand you happiness on a silver platter. Learn the Divine Spiritual Wisdom and serve others so that you may be both a liberator and liberated.

When you begin to walk the path of our Divine Spiritual Wisdom, you join others on a path of divinity, service, and uplifting others, for we are walking within the framework of Godhood. The practice of our Divine Spiritual Wisdom bestows consciousness and intelligence. To serve others, you must have power. When the conscious and intelligent believe that everything comes from God and consistently serve others, they become trouble free. Therefore, forget your own concerns and go out of your way to serve all those who cross your path. As you do so, you will be rewarded; when you heal another's problems, your own will disappear. Problems only arise when we are not doing our part to take care of others.

Serve others, for through service, Eve, our fallen soul, becomes "Mary", our rising soul. When you are more concerned with taking than serving, you enslave your soul. As a result, you lose contact with the higher world. This time corresponds to the coming of a Christos, and in this Age it is imperative that we face the regeneration of Eve through service to others. In this way we will be able to go to war with the Dragon and more easily face "Mary," the water of regeneration, so that we may purify the world. Our sacred science allows you to understand that serving others is the highest form of Kabbalah. It is the highest form of yoga. It is the heavenly act of giving light, for where there is light, you cannot find darkness, and darkness cannot remain in the presence of light. As you give light to others, the universe gives you light in the form of a deep healing joy. Presently, the culture of our society is quite individualistic, most people are takers, not givers. Incidentally, all you have to do to find out whether a person is a taker or giver, is to look at the shape of their upper and lower lips. Those who take and do not give in equal measure disrupt their internal balance. In other words, the balance of give and take is lost within those who take more than they give. They are then subject to illnesses that are reflective of this imbalance. For example, cancer is a disease in which the affected cells become selfish and will not share.

In another example, you will notice that many wealthy people suffer from heart attacks, for they have not given in proportion to what they have received. In this case, bring the tip of the index finger on the Venus mount (at the base of the thumb), and join the tips of the middle and ring fingers to the tips of the thumbs, so they are placed side by side. The little finger remaining straight, meditate with the *Heaven's Touch* or *Sounds of the Ether* CDs to cure or prevent heart attack or heart problems.

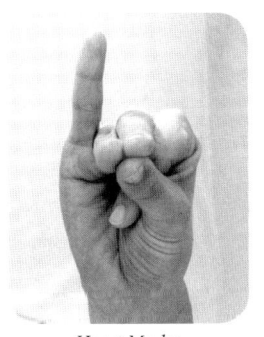

Heart Mudra

Human beings must learn to share with others. We must become like the sun, that heavenly body that shines its light indiscriminately on all of the earth's inhabitants. Sharing is what the Universe understands. Therefore, when we create lives of service and sharing, the Universe responds to us positively. What we all need to realize, however, is that serving others brings the healing joy of life. Whoever truly experiences such joy finds that it not only heals a person, but it also fills the heart and soul to the brim. It matters not if the creature comforts or status of this world elude him, for the light of his kindness, the sympathy attendant with his growing love for humanity, the virtue that springs forth from his heart, these qualities enlighten and enliven his soul. The end goal of Kabbalah, yoga, and all form of mysticism and healing, is to be a better servant to humanity. All that we experience, from the beginning of the spiritual journey to the end, trains us to be better able to serve mankind. Understand that if this is not the intention of the person, he will find that in the end he has accomplished nothing. Again, it is only by treading along the path of service to others that our souls can rise up from the lowest depths to the highest heaven. The fare to gain entry into the higher, heavenly realm is knowledge of the Divine Spiritual Wisdom and service, and the higher one evolves, the more he/she desires to serve. The most liberating action is to serve others. Indeed, those who are of a higher evolution are ready and willing to console with their words, lend a sympathetic ear, and help through their deeds. Go out of your way to serve those who cross your path. In this way, you will become increasingly like a heavenly rose whose fragrance is both healing and uplifting.

Learn the laws of nature contained in Universal Kabbalah and serve others. The most important moment of any act is its beginning moment, because the beginning moment sets the stage for the future. Start a marriage, business, or project at an inauspicious time, and it will always carry a negative vibration, which will cause you to be miserable or experience health challenges. Start a marriage, business, or project at the right time, and the beneficial forces of nature will strive to give you happiness and the very best. It is by knowing and working with the laws of nature that we are able to determine when to initiate something new in our lives. Remember, the manner in which something is begun determines whether or not it will bring happiness or sorrow. Therefore, it is vital that you learn the laws of nature contained in Universal Kabbalah. This knowledge will give you light, and the light will take care of you. Even if you do not believe in God, you cannot deny the fact that there is an order in nature. God does all according to law. He works in mysterious ways to perform His wonders. When man undertakes learning the

Divine Spiritual Wisdom, he begins to recognize the perfection of the organization of the universe as God created it. If we wish to be connected with God, and be considered one of His servants, we must truly comprehend and respect the laws that God created for us to follow. Otherwise, we are but walking corpses. Our soul was designed by God to be liberated, and help us achieve a glorious existence, but our negligence of the divine laws and our forgetfulness that He is in everything, has resulted in a global existence that is devoid of deeper meaning and is fraught with turmoil.

The laws of nature guide our entire lives. We live and die and are born again by these laws. They are the basis of our world and our very being; from them all wisdom can be plucked like ripe fruit for the eating. The laws of nature are eternal signposts. They were there yesterday, they are here today, and they will be there tomorrow, guiding human beings to yield. Unfortunately, most do not heed their pronouncements and life becomes progressively miserable. As human beings we have two choices. We can either fight the laws of nature, or flow with them. When we flow with them, we bring ourselves into harmony with the whole universe and the universe serves us. In other words, when you flow in harmony with the laws of nature, the Infinite takes care of you, completely and totally, in each and every moment.

The *Alchemy of Love Relationships, The Divine Doctor*, and *Lifting the Veil*, are three books that will be of great benefit as you journey through this life. Each assists with a different aspect of earthly existence. The first of the three reveals the laws of love. The second reveals the laws of health and the importance of self-healing. The third reveals the laws of life and will help you gain transcendence of perception as you move through time and space. The *Self Study Course* is also available. It delves more deeply into these subjects while bestowing further knowledge. And finally, the *Akashic Record*, which was developed from some of the natural and universal laws outlined in the three books mentioned as well as the *Self Study Course*, will guide you on your way. Working with our teachings will cause you to start using powers that have been asleep for your entire life. The Divine Spiritual Wisdom from Universal Kabbalah contained in these books and self-study course, will take care of your mental, emotional, and physical health. It teaches you the truth of the universe, and that truth is simple, pure, and clear. By giving you the key to all mysteries and a full knowledge of the inner workings of nature and creation, you develop the capacity to see and know those things that others cannot see and do not yet know. In comparison with the majority of people who pursue spiritual understanding, you will be one of the few who have gained access to true spiritual methodology. Even those who obediently pray, meditate, and endeavor to live spiritual lives will never grasp the greater truths of the universe if they cannot comprehend the laws that govern every aspect of human life. Never rush madly into something without first seeking God's blessing through an understanding of His laws. It is imperative that you know the laws of nature and ask for God's blessing before undertaking anything.

For God's sake, be a good spiritual lawyer. Know the laws of nature before trying to break them. Always know where you are going, and you will not get lost along the way. There is a place for each of us in this world, but it is our job to discover it. We do not have to search the world over for our happiness or our life's purpose. All we need to do is work on ourselves using the Naam, and apply the laws of nature outlined in Universal Kabbalah. Universal Kabbalah is the purest and safest method of walking the spiritual path, for the path of Universal Kabbalah is the path of the Sun and service. Fear-based dogma, apparent in other spiritual and/or religious practices, is not found in Universal Kabbalah. You will find that those who work with the Divine Spiritual Wisdom have a luminous, magnetic, and beautiful aura. Universal Kabbalists are bright, warm, and radiant like the sun, and are surrounded and protected by the Christic shield of Lumen de Lumine. At the very moment that you begin to learn our sacred science, practice with the Word, and serve others, the destiny written on your forehead changes. This is called the law of meridian change. Universal Kabbalah will lift the veil that blankets your soul, and give you a clearer vision of your life's purpose, your reason for being here on earth. It will synchronize your mind and heart in praise of the Lord, and you will be touched by His vastness. As it cleanses your mind of negativity, opens your eyes, deeply touches your heart, and awakens your soul, the opportunities that perfectly suit you will arise. Moreover, you will see the light of your soul, which will cast its beam far and wide, enabling you to see the indescribable wonder of God, nature, and man.

If you want to acquire knowledge of the divine spiritual sciences, begin our self-study course. Indeed, the Divine Spiritual Wisdom contained in this course will not only heal you, but will also spiritualize, enhance, and embellish your life, making it absolutely Divine. Those who follow the divine spiritual teachings can be assured of learning the purest, fastest and most direct path to the eternal truths. Learning the Divine Spiritual Wisdom is the key to understanding the language of heaven and earth. It is the language of the angelic, or celestial beings.

Hermes Mercurius Trismegistus, the Three Times Great, was the wisest Egyptian priest, and known as the father of the Divine Spiritual Wisdom. The ancient Egyptians regarded him as the embodiment of the Universal Mind. Hermes was a supreme philosopher with vast knowledge, a supreme priest in his holiness of life and practice of divine cults, and a supreme administrator of the laws worthy of kingly dignity. All fundamental and basic teachings embedded in the esoteric teachings of every race can be traced back to this Master of all arts, sciences, and crafts, this Ruler of the Three Worlds, Scribe of the Gods, and Keeper of the Books of Life. With these sacred teachings, you will learn to know God, nature, and man.

Our lineage descends from Adam to Noah, from Noah to Melchisedek, and on to Abraham, Moses, Saul, David, Solomon, Zerubbabel, and Christ. The one who pointed the way to Jesus the Christ, was Moses, son of Amram and Jochebed, from the tribe of Levi, and younger brother of Miriam and Aaron. Adopted by an Egyptian princess, Moses lived in Egypt for many years. At God's command, he parted the Red Sea, creating an escape route for the Israelites as they fled the Egyptian army. Moses received the Ten Commandments from God, written on two stone tablets, on Mount Sinai, and is credited with writing the first five books of the Bible. Christ is the Active, Intelligent Cause, the Great Chief and Guide to whom the order of the universe has been committed until a time when man, now in a state of separation, has been reconciled with the One and only Source. This universal order was originally entrusted to mankind before the fall; now, we are under Christ's aegis until we may regain our rightful place in the universe. We follow the Christic path, believing in the immortality of the soul and in its final reintegration. We are friends of heaven, and an extension of God here on earth, chosen by the Father to follow his Son in the Light of the holy spirit in order to remember the truth of the holy scriptures. We pursue the knowledge contained within the Divine Spiritual Wisdom that transports the body and soul to the highest glory of the Creator. As Universal Kabbalists, we believe in God who has made the heavens and earth, and to whom we pledge unconditional loyalty; for our strength, power, and graces come from Him, and recognize Christ as the Word made flesh, along with the holy scriptures. We serve and love others with neutrality with no expectation that the love will be returned. We participate actively in sharing the Divine Spiritual Wisdom to help lighten the burdens of others, and awaken the love of the great Architect of the Universe in their hearts. For He is the One giving us will, strength and power to face the challenges of time and space gracefully. We use love, faith, hope, forgiveness, and charity in our sacred work.

Our path is the path of prayer—the bread of the soul. We pray to learn how to pray better, not only for us, but above all, for other beings. We pray so that we may become a clear channel through which the light of God may enter the hearts of others so as to melt away darkness for good. We pray that the Creator can see it fit to grace our lives with His Omnipresence, Omniscience and Omnipower so we may work for his glory on this planet earth. Our sacred teachings originate with the Creator himself, and have been perpetuated since the days of Adam. We belong to the Community of the Elect of Light, which grants us the nourishing fire of strength to act upon everything in nature. We possess the key that opens the gate of mystery. Our Word, touch, presence and blessings bring the entire psyche and being of a person into balance, for we know that we are connected with the Higher Worlds, and that the union of the will with Divinity makes the marvels of nature subordinate to us. We invite you to join this Community of Light in which the Spirit of Wisdom itself will guide and teach all who approach with a genuine thirst for knowledge. Under Its tutelage, Divinity bends to mankind so that it may write the Truth in our souls, the Truth that is an eternal mystery. All one needs to be a servant of the universe is to be humble, simple like a little child, charitable, loving towards your neighbor, and forgiving of your enemies.

Those who join the self-study course will learn how to create the purest line of contact with helpful angelic entities. Joining this course will give you all the tools you need to be a true lighthouse, so that you may experience self-healing, and serve others. It cannot be stressed enough that this sacred work is for those who seek the Truth with a good and honest heart. We must rediscover our Divine Nature so that we may celebrate Love, Light and Freedom within us all. The spiritual wisdom contained in the Universal Kabbalah self-study course ignites the Mysterium Conjunctionis of the Alchemists within you, which is symbolized by the Star of David that unites the upper heavenly triangle with the lower earthly triangle. By working with this sacred course you will experience the indescribable joy and ecstatic bliss that comes from the true spiritual marriage born from the merger of heaven and earth. The course causes the Holy Spirit to spiritualize matter so that you may see the light of the soul, which will bring the harmony of heaven in your life. This sacred work will turn your body into a perfect temple for the Holy Ghost, leading to health, wholeness and harmony. Learn to work with the wisdom of the Ages to affect positive Planetary Transformation. Learn the Divine Spiritual Wisdom contained in Universal Kabbalah, so that you may romance with God, and the entire universe will serve you. Feel His tender kiss and become blissful, radiant, and beautiful. Learn these sacred teachings and work with the Word so that they may root your being firmly in the soil of the soul and allow you to partake of the fruit of ecstasy. Let their healing waves melt the darkness in your life away so that you are able to dance with the Angels. Learning the Divine Spiritual Wisdom is the key to understanding the language of heaven and earth. He who masters the elegance, logic, and beauty of the Divine Spiritual Wisdom contained in Universal Kabbalah, is able to converse with God's messengers. Thus, when you work with these sacred teachings, you receive the blessings of the Holy Angels, Archangels, Virtues, Powers, Thrones, Dominations, Cherubim, and Seraphim.

*From the beginning of time through the very confines
of prehistoric days to present day,
we find the influence of the seven creative planets
governed by these seven Archangels.
These Archangels direct and control the entire course
of life through the seven planetary bodies.
This mysterious energetic influence affects every
sentient being in the universe.
The seven planets not only compose the karmic wheel;
they set in motion the universal laws that are
responsible for the order and regularity of
everything in Heaven and on Earth.
They ensure that we comply with the natural laws,
systems and order of things in the universe
to which we owe our very Being.*

15

THE SEVEN ARCHANGELS

There is a Divine Code in the universe comprised of the laws of the main Archangels who stand before the throne of God and whose magnetic influence operates through the creative planets, radiating over the Earth. This Divine Code is the system Mother Nature uses in Her mysterious dealings with life. Having knowledge of this Code is like possessing a Master Key that unlocks the mysteries of Heaven and Earth. It can help you take care of your health, nurture your love life, and gain success in your career. Divine truth comes through the laws of nature. The Law of the seven Archangels is part of the same laws that guide the trees in their growth, and make the poppies close at night and open each morning. These laws are not religious. They are Divine and universal because God created them. The faster you come into harmony with the Divine, universal laws of nature, the faster you will be in harmony and your life will change. Working with the Divine Spiritual Wisdom will cause you to leave your doubts, fears, sorrows, and skepticism, behind. Having healed yourself of such negativity, you will find that happiness, confidence, and harmony take their place. The word law connotes power and control. It is the rule of law that makes the universe so entirely dependable. This dependability, evident in the sun's daily rise above the horizon, allows human beings to plan a calendar a century in advance, predict eclipses of the Sun and Moon with accuracy, and chart a schedule of the ocean's tides. Indeed, natural and universal law allow for the very life and growth of the planet and its inhabitants. If we accept that natural and universal law is the cornerstone of the universe, it follows that the same law governs every phase of human development. When we study natural and universal law, we gain knowledge, power, and wisdom. The universe is ruled by laws which never change. Knowing and understanding the laws of life releases us from fear, for within these laws lie the tools that aid us in creating something beautiful with our lives. All we need to do is utilize the principles that have been discovered and tested by our sages. In so doing we honor nature. Remember, when you follow these laws and commit to serving others, you are on the road that leads to success, health, and joy. Those who fail to pay their obligations will see their joy, happiness, and opportunities to serve diminish. Similarly, those who cause others pain, sorrow, misery, and anxiety will, through the principle of causality, reap the very same qualities of emotion, for nature works and manifests through exact, infinite, and ever-perfect laws, rules, and operations. Violate the laws and nature will not only rebuke you, She will repay you in kind with the precise gradation of unhappiness you have caused. In other words, he who transgresses will experience similar transgressions somewhere in life. Now is the time for the greater truths concerning the nature of these laws at this moment in history to be shared and expanded upon throughout the world. Moreover, the Divine has ordained their usage so that the promise of great transformation can be brought about exactly at this time; we have held this space in time for worldwide healing since the beginning of ages past. All you need to do is make living in accordance with Divine Law your highest priority in life.

The great hidden truth contained in the operation of the seven Archangels, who stand for the expression of the mysterious God force in nature, may forever remain a mystery to those who have not yet realized the importance of the Divine Spiritual Wisdom.

Each soul that is born is an emanation from the Great Spiritual Being that rules the universe and is referred to in the bible as the Elohim, or the seven Archangels of the presence, which rule the signs of the zodiac through the planets. Every one of the planets ruled by the Archangels bring upon the soul the varying experiences, joys, temptations, and testing which a careful study of the greater map of the heavens will elucidate and make clear. From the beginning of time this great clock of the heavens has marked off its hours, and planetary rulers, the regent of the stars, have passed in grand procession with the light of their inimitable illumination through the pathway marked out. The seven Archangels are the seven avenues through which the Sun of righteousness, the incarnate Word, can shine forth and illuminate the hearts and minds of all classes and conditions of humanity. They stand for the seven Elohim, expressed through the seven nature notes and the seven colors into which the one white light (or the Yod) is broken up. Also, they represent the seven gates to the new Jerusalem, that inner temple of truth in which each human can receive the illumination of the inner mysteries, face to face and heart to heart through his own special avenues of thought and teachings. That inner shrine where the One light reveals those inner truths which cannot be given directly to the uncomprehended multitude, but which are the basis of the outer shining forth of every true disciple of the Christ force. Jesus Christ fed the multitude with five loaves and two small fish, and with the remaining fragments he gathered twelve baskets full. These seven cervical vertebrae stand for the forces of five exoteric planets and the two esoteric planets hidden behind the Sun and the Moon. And these seven planetary forces must be recognized and assimilated so that one can fill the baskets with the forces of those planets expressed through the twelve thoracic vertebrae and symbolized by the twelve signs of the zodiac. The planetary rulers of the seven sacred powers, or Creative Forces of the Cosmos, govern the kingdoms of the macrocosm and manifest in the twelve divisions of the celestial zodiac.

Divine justice operates through these seven Archangels and uses the seven creative planets, which compose the karmic wheel to restore harmony in all things. After King Solomon, son of King David, ascended to the throne and the knowledge and wisdom he so fervently desired was bestowed upon him by the Creator, he said: "I thank thee O Creator of the universe that thou has taught me the secrets of the planets that I may knowest the times and seasons of things; the secrets of men's hearts, their thoughts, and the nature of their Being, thou gavest unto me this knowledge which is the foundation of all my wisdom." It is that same secret understanding of the nature of the seven planets that allows us to determine some of what the future may hold. And that same secret reveals that the seven creative planets which correspond to the seven Archangels who sit before the throne of God and whose magnetic influence radiates over the Earth, affect our health, love relationship, career and happiness in general. Those who have mastered that sacred science already know how to move through life gracefully. In actuality, the seven creative planets have been the outcome of the influence of the seven Archangels, who sit before the throne of God. They are also responsible for the seven days of the week, which exist throughout the world. It is written in the Zohar, seven lights are there in the most high, and there dwell the most ancients, the secret of secrets, the hidden of all hidden ones—Ain Soph. The magnetic influence of the seven Archangels who stand forever before the throne, have helped the laws of God become known on this earth long before human made his creeds and man made laws.

From the beginning of time through the very confines of prehistoric days to present day, we find the influence of the seven creative planets governed by these seven Archangels in every country of the world. These Archangels direct and control the entire course of life through the seven planetary bodies. This mysterious energetic influence affects every sentient being in the universe. The seven planets not only compose the karmic wheel; they set in motion the universal laws that are responsible for the order and regularity of everything in Heaven and on Earth. They ensure that we comply with the natural laws, systems and order of things in the universe to which we owe our very Being.

Everything on Earth and in Heaven contains meaning, especially its secret and soul meaning, as well as its place and number in the order of things, as decreed in the Heavenly design. Every day of the week, every hour of the day has a corresponding sacred meaning and number that governs its action, attesting to the incredible regularity and organization of Heaven, which is beyond word. The Sun, Jupiter, and Venus are beneficent planets whereas Mars and Saturn are challenging planets. The Moon and Mercury remain neutral, so they can go either way.

You need only experiment with the seven creative planets for a few months, when you will be forced to notice how easily things turn for you during your Sun, Jupiter and Venus periods. You will be struck with the strong fact that under these three beneficial periods, things will be favorable for your plan or business and you will display much more magnetism during these periods of the year. You will notice too that the same law applies to your own vitality and health. How you have felt "down" at certain periods of the year, which you will also notice come regularly when you have not been within the favorable period indicated for you.

If you are open minded you will begin to apply this knowledge to all your actions. You will no longer make appointments at random. You will then begin to notice how much easier the machinery of your affairs works, you will no longer lose your head or be frightened when worries appear to come from every side. You can then expect challenges at certain periods and make your plans accordingly. In a short time you will notice how much more successful you have become and how, with less effort in every sense, more can be accomplished.

You will then begin to apply the same rules to your home. You will no longer be as fearful and anxious when you feel there is nothing to guide you. You will know when to expect those moments of depression and vulnerability when your love relationship is going through challenges. You will no longer seek solace in drugs, smoking, alcohol or bars. God who controls each millisecond of time and the movements of millions of the world's processes, regulates also the action of humans. To the most unsuccessful this blueprint will bring success. To those who are already successful, it will bring health and higher opportunities for them to experience their vastness.

By a hidden law of destiny over which man has no control, President Bush was in his Mars period and Senator Kerry in his Saturn period, during the election day within a cosmic time period where Uranus casts it presence. When you bring together Mars and Saturn and Uranus during a waning moon, a challenging event takes place. Mars and Saturn are the two most challenging planets known in the entire spiritual kingdom. This is why the country was so divided, and predicting the outcome of that particular election appears to be so difficult. Mars and Saturn are two of the seven creative planets which correspond to the seven Archangels who sit before the throne of God and whose magnetic influence radiates over the Earth. They initiate the karmic wheel.

Turning to the more mysterious or hidden influences indicated by Mars and Saturn, they have a most peculiar spiritual symbolism, giving clear warning of a strange challenge. Saturn and Mars are also symbolic of the unknown, the unexpected, cautioning prudence and patience. Therefore one should pray to avert their fatalistic tendencies when under the influence of these two planets. The presence of Uranus in this Age of the glory of self, increases the fatalistic indication given by Mars and Saturn.

The spiritual symbolism of Saturn is represented by the figure of justice, with a sword pointing upwards and a balance or scales in the left hand. It is mainly characterized by difficulty, delay and obstacles. Saturn is the symbol of mystery, which causes the people it rules to be misunderstood. They work hard and strive earnestly to carry out their dream, yet their plans usually meet with opposition. However, if they spend time developing their spiritual side, people ruled by Saturn can overcome any challenge, making the impossible possible. Mars is personified as a strong masculine figure dressed as a warrior and riding a ram. Mars is the symbol of war and power, which, if wrongly used, will bring destruction. Both the job of Mars, the lord of war, and Saturn, the Lord of Karma, is to create karmic balance through challenging circumstances. Therefore, these two presidential candidates had to overcome enormous challenges. Although these two planets are challenging, you will find that most successful people have Mars for determination, and/or Saturn for discipline. Mars and Saturn are seen as challenging planets but in reality they can be favorable, you just need to know how to work with them. Each person receives the influence of Mars and Saturn differently. Therefore, each person will experience their effects differently. The primary objective of Mars and Saturn is to rid us of all impurity and disharmony. In other words, their role is to cleanse and purify. If one is unable to handle such purification, he/she will be challenged. Indeed, while the initiate who knows how to transform can experience Mars and Saturn as propitious, the uninitiated will be upset by their influence. Kindness, love, and gentleness are needed to counteract Mars and Saturn. When you are serious about working for good, all planets, including Mars and Saturn, become beneficial. Raise your consciousness, your frequency, and you will be able to successfully handle Mars and Saturn. You will no longer be bound by the rules of the dualistic world. You will approach the Sun, which is the One.

Challenges, or hard luck, which are the activity of Saturn or Mars, are a manifestation of a law over which one has no control. Conversely, good luck, or the activity of the Sun (fame), Jupiter (glory and wealth) or Venus (love) is the manifestation of the law that causes personal convenience. In Universal Kabbalah you will learn that each one of us has a primary, secondary, tertiary, quaternary, quinary, senary, and septenary planet that combine to determine the blessings and challenges that we will grow through from our first breath to our last. In other words, human beings have a combination of planets that govern their existence, giving them blessings and obstacles so that they may develop their spirituality.

A spiritual law dictates that the application of any given force affects all the orders in the object to which it is applied, whichever of those orders is directly affected. This indicates that the spiritual seeds planted during the election of the United States, which is the leading country of the world, will affect everyone on earth. Since we are all interconnected and live on one earth, this election affects not only the United States, but the whole planet. It represents the seed of an event that will produce a tree in 2012. Seeding is one of the greatest principles of the Rose Croix Kabbalists; the seed is a germ or power from which a being grows. A seed represents the birth or blossoming of a force within the world. Everything is in the seed. There are seeds of elementals, minerals, plants, animals, and humans. In Kabbalah the seed is called *Aleph*. It is the beginning. The beginning controls the end. All your power is at the beginning of an action. The important thing here is that the electoral process which is the seed of the event took place for President Bush and Senator Kerry, while they are respectively in their Mars and Saturn periods. This took place while there were their karmic periods, at a karmic time. The beginning determines the end. If you cannot see the tree in the seed, you cannot see God in this world. The beginning of an act is the most important moment of all. For it allows you to know the nature of the forces that are being triggered and the consequences that will follow from the action undertaken.

Many have written to ask how to mitigate and transform the influence of a fatalistic planet in their lives. In truth, the universe is governed by immutable laws. The law of the seven Archangels are immutable cosmic laws that are final and entirely different from man made laws and operate on an unknown plane. God, the great Architect of the universe, effected the manifestation of certain laws so they might operate towards a certain end. In our limited ability to understand these laws, we are even more limited in our ability to perceive their outcome since we can only comprehend a fraction of the original intelligence, God, who instituted these principles.

People give little thought to their place in the universe, or are seldom conscious of the manifestation of the laws of the seven Archangels, unless these laws interrupt their human lives or create an inward crisis that brings them to their attention. It is important to keep in mind that we live in a purposeful universe governed by a superior intelligence. And the law of the seven Archangels is a cosmic and absolutely just law that is immutable until the purpose is fulfilled. Divine justice is indicated by the fact that the law of the seven Archangels operating through the seven creative planets will continue to operate towards their end whether or not every man and woman understands them or even works with them. One cannot change the laws of the seven Archangels, because they work for a purpose which is much more important and much more significant in the entire cosmic scheme than our little selves.

Most people have to work hard, constantly struggling to get just a few of the things that this earthly life has to offer. Vibrating the Word and working with the laws of the seven Archangels, can help make life less of a struggle and, therefore, more enjoyable. The laws of the seven Archangels, based on the highly secret and mystical Divine Spiritual Wisdom known as Universal Kabbalah, are the most powerful, beneficial, and protective tools of all time. When you apply the Divine Spiritual Wisdom and work with the Word, you cause the beneficial forces of the universe to act in your best interest by protecting you from danger and misfortune, and helping you achieve a productive, satisfying earthly life. Learning and applying the Divine Spiritual Wisdom while working with the Word is a cosmic key that has the power to open the doors of opportunity, remove obstacles, and help you achieve the realization of your dreams and ambitions. Indeed, those who apply the Divine Spiritual Wisdom and work with the Word receive a shower of heavenly blessings and live lives of divine angelic help, guidance, and protection.

Human beings are created in material form with Divine power and energy. This enables us to appreciate and honor all that God provides in nature, and to return a portion of what we have been given through good deeds and uplifting words. God gave man the ability, the power, and the energy to utilize the products of nature to maintain life. Although He gave us the first breath of life, we must earn every breath thereafter. In exchange for the life force that God placed in man, we must give back to nature an equal amount of force, or energy. According to the Law, as man compensates nature, so shall nature compensate man. As we give to nature with respect to the order of the universe by working with the laws of the seven Archangels, nature will compensate us. If at any time, however, we fail to carry out our obligations to nature, we will be made to compensate for our dereliction of duty through suffering. Think of it this way, you can compensate willingly by working with the laws of the seven Archangels, or you can be compelled to compensate through suffering. Should you choose the path of working against the forces of nature, you will not only be made to suffer, you may pass on without enjoying the true happiness and joy that could have been yours. The laws will continue to keep the universe in order and compensate those who work with them.

The Universal Kabbalist strives to maintain good health, and is aware that the key to good health lies in obedience to the laws of nature. When faced with challenging mental, emotional, or physical states of being, the Universal Kabbalist remains steady in his/her attunement with the universe and adherence to living in harmony with natural and spiritual laws. In this way, he/she can invoke heavenly help in whatever he/she wishes to accomplish. Furthermore, in living in such a manner, the Universal Kabbalist is recognized for the positive and uplifting vibrations he/she radiates, for he/she has developed the strength and courage necessary to manifest only that which is in tune with the infinite. The Universal Kabbalist is alive with the purifying, vitalizing, healing forces of the universe to such an extent that his/her life becomes an expression of strength, serenity, prosperity, and health. In turn, his/her vision becomes clearer, his/her heart happier, and his/her person richer in numerous ways.

We highly recommend that those who wish to receive divine protection from negative forces, bad luck, and misfortune, including all physical and spiritual attacks, work with the law of the seven Archangels and vibrate the Word. Think for a moment how many people might benefit from these sacred teachings. Think of the joy, the comfort, and the hope that would blossom and grow in many hearts and souls by reconnecting with the Divine Spiritual Wisdom. The happiness that these teachings inspire is the birthright of every living being.

You can work with the law of the seven Archangels to improve your health, your love relationship, and your life. These are fully covered in the books: *The Divine Doctor, Alchemy of Love Relationships,* and *Lifting the Veil.* The manifestation of the law of the seven Archangels affects everyone. They are the reason why the universe moves in such order and harmony. They are not only the ruling laws of this Age, but they will also be visibly active in our lives to 2012 and beyond. When we work to understand them, we automatically receive help from Heaven. Therefore, if we have gained an insight that makes it possible for us to enter into a deeper relationship with these laws, then we must compensate for the benefits that we have gained. For example, if we are fortunate in business, money matters, or health, then we should strive through our own effort of sharing our gains to make it possible to truly assist others who are not as fortunate, and who desire similar goals as ours. It is important to remember that we are all interconnected throughout the whole universe. We should stop acting as if we are separate from one another. By serving others we are helping ourselves.

The other thing to keep in mind is that the presence of the two pentagrams in October 2004, right before the presidential election, brought to light the importance of the Christic mysteries. These events will affect us for the many years to come. They presage the fact that there is a new and great force emerging in our world, a force that evokes the Christic energy that lives within our very souls, and which manifests in all the great and wonderful occurrences of our lives.

16

OUR PLANETARY BODIES

As a human soul incarnates lifetime after lifetime, it resonates with a certain planetary combination that bestows dominant characteristics. In the course of the soul's journey through matter it takes on a physical body, and the individual is born under the influence of various planetary conditions. It is possible, then, for human beings, composed as we are of the essences of all of the planetary bodies, to succeed in becoming superior to any combination of planetary bodies. In order for any one of us to be victorious over the planetary influences, however, we must pass through the seven Archangels and master the influences of the planetary bodies they govern—a process which may require numerous incarnations. Only when a man or woman has gathered within all that the planetary forces hold for him/her, can it be said that he/she is one of the Elect. In the course of a specific incarnation, the soul incarnates under a particular vibration, ruled by a combination of planetary bodies, in order to learn the lessons particular to the degree of manifestation of that force. The Creator constructed human beings according to a definite plan, creating distinct types of people ruled by primary, secondary, tertiary, quaternary, and quinary planets. Each of the five planetary bodies attributed to the individual reveal certain qualities, aptitudes, virtues, and faults, as well as peculiarities of health and character. While it may seem strange that such disparate types were created, the combination of qualities represented by the planetary bodies attributed to each of us is absolutely necessary for the harmonious operation of the universe. After the individual has passed through an incarnation in a particular combination of planetary bodies, learning as much or as little as he can, he incarnates in another combination. Upon doing so, he carries with him all the experience gained from the previous planetary combination. Built into his new body, then, are inherent faculties and abilities. This process continues until the individual has moved through the various combinations to mastery. As the individual returns to the original combination of planetary bodies, he/she has added powers. He/she can now resume the same lessons on a higher plane and with a greater power to manifest the positive forces of that particular combination.

Many people wander aimlessly through life, never settling down because they have not found their true place. They have not found the work, love relationship, and lifestyle that suits them best. Rootless and unhappy, they are like seeds waiting to be put into fertile ground so that they can germinate. Happiness eludes you if you do not know where your true place is. *"Know thyself, and thou wilt know the Universe of the Gods."* Know yourself, and you then know the planets, the "gods" of all celestial bodies, which are the brain of heaven. The five planets that comprise your planetary blueprint allow you to know yourself, your strengths and weaknesses, so that you are able to recognize your own personal fertile ground, the place where you can be sown and blossom into a beautiful flower. You determine your future every day, every hour and every minute. Knowing your five planets sets you instantly on the path of light. Your planetary blueprint reveals your character. When you learn about your five planets, you gain knowledge of who you truly are. Similarly, when you learn about the five planets of friends and loved ones, you gain knowledge of who they truly are. Such knowledge of self and others can help you to be of service in your relationships. In some instances, knowledge of the five planets enables you to foretell what may happen in the future, because it gives you the clues that allow for clarity. By working with the positive aspects of your five planetary bodies, you activate beneficial forces within. In turn, these forces eventually act favorably on those around you. The object of creation is to evolve and redeem every atom of the planet. Man will never complete this task, however, until he has discovered the Divine Harmony of the Hierarchy to which he belongs. Understand that miracles are revealed through man in God's image. Learning these sacred teachings will put hope in our souls, faith in our spirits, and love in our hearts, as we are able to see the beauty and light of life. Then, the entirety of heaven speaks to us, for we are in direct communication with the invisible world. At this time, it is our responsibility to infuse the harmonious force of love and perfection we encounter into our environment, beginning with our own bodies and moving on to each and every kingdom of animal, plant, mineral, and particle of matter we can touch through our healing thought waves.

Knowledge of the five planetary bodies particular to our present incarnation enables us to probe more deeply into our inner nature, so that we may understand ourselves completely. Once this step has taken place, we are released from unconscious compulsions and motivations, and we may truly begin to gain spiritual mastery over our lives. This process causes us to fully express our inner self in everyday activities, as well as be attuned to our destiny in the divine plan. In essence, your planetary bodies allow you to fortify various areas within your life in preparation for what is to come in the future, and align you so that you are more capable of being a successful conduit for constructive energies. You cannot deny that these planetary bodies are part of you, part of the feelings that formulate your character and your personality. They must be explored and understood so that you can gain time and space, and express yourself in a natural way. Understand them so that you are able to understand yourself and be the human being that you truly are. Allow this understanding to guide you to a neutral space of your own Divinity so that you can achieve clarity. In other words, allow yourself to be both human and Divine through an understanding of these planets.

The salvation of man lies in his capacity to concentrate on the Divine Spiritual Wisdom, for this capacity allows him to walk forever peacefully on the path of light. In this age, we must work with this sacred science to heal ourselves, help others, and contribute to a positive evolution of humankind, for we are all interconnected and a reflection of each other. We do not have to be bound by the actions of our past. Instead, we can choose to act utilizing the knowledge of the laws of nature in the present as if we were a new person, reformed by the Divine Spiritual Wisdom, which is designed to make our journey through life happy, successful, and fulfilling.

Tenth Body Meditation

Position:
Sit straight in easy pose with a straight spine. Cross the wrists at 90 degrees, 10 inches from the nose, palms open to the face at eye level, right wrist in front of left. Keep thumbs in line with the hand, wrist, and forearm.

Mantra:
Inhale deeply and chant the *Guru Gaitri Mantra* three times in one breath. (Optional: chant along with *The Flow of Naam* CD.)

Gobinday	*(Sustainer)*
Mukunday	*(Liberator)*
Udaray	*(Enlightener)*
Aparay	*(Infinite)*
Hariang	*(Destroyer)*
Kariang	*(Creator)*
Nirnamay	*(Nameless)*
Akamay	*(Desireless)*

Time:
Continue for 11 minutes, chanting rhythmically and rapidly. To end, inhale deeply and hold the breath for 5-10 seconds, then relax.

Comments:
When you have truly merged with the Divine Spiritual Wisdom, and connected with the spirit of God in you, you become fully satisfied and complete within yourself. In your oneness with God, you see that the whole universe is ready to serve you. The mantra describes God in various aspects. By chanting this mantra in this mudra 11,000 times, one can avoid a prewritten death, manifest any positive wish, and erase any negativity in one's personal destiny.

17

THE POWER OF SACRED MUSIC

THERE IS NOTHING MORE IMPORTANT as a means of healing the human body through the soul, and nothing that can be of greater use and importance on the path of spiritual attainment, than sacred music. As every word that comes out of one's mouth has its effect not only upon one's body, but also upon one's mind and spirit, so can the kind of music one hears heal and prove to be of great advantage to oneself. Working with sacred music or the music of the soul, is not only a medical process of consciousness, but also, it is a psycho therapy that enables you to get rid of sickness.

The medical community is now coming to the understanding that sacred music can be used to effectively manage pain, moods, depression, blood pressure, and anxiety, as well as the nausea associated with chemotherapy and the immobility associated with Parkinson's disease. Indeed, exciting research suggests that the brain responds to music almost as if it were medicine. The anecdotal evidence of music therapists bolsters the credibility of such research by demonstrating that the healing properties of music can lessen a patient's post-surgery recovery time while helping them handle future complications. Many in the field recommend that music be used in conjunction with traditional healing modalities. To this end, the Rootlight Sacred Music series can do much to help patients, as it creates a positive, uplifting atmosphere in which they are better able to cope with the health challenges they face. Our sacred music warms the heart, soothes the soul, and stimulates concentration and creativity.

Sound is not only beneficial in times of physical distress and challenged health, but also, music affects development in the womb and in early childhood. Researchers observe an increase in fetal heart rate when in the presence of music. Moreover, when a mother listens to sacred music during her pregnancy, she creates a healing, soothing, and uplifting environment for the child to enter into. Of course, a child continues to develop after birth, when environment and experience combine to create mental circuits and patterns between neurons, those electrically charged nerve cells that transfer information through the brain. When the neurons are not exercised, they cease to properly form the necessary pathways. The brain then trims the fat, so to speak, by pruning the unused neurons. Understand that a critical window of opportunity for the development of both verbal and musical abilities opens at birth and closes around the age of eleven. Music can assist in the cognitive development of very young children, for musical training generates the neural connections used during abstract reasoning and the assimilation of mathematical concepts. Meanwhile, the spoken language heard by an infant creates a complex set of interconnections that have an important impact on overall brain development. To be sure, there is an overlap in the neurons used to process music, language, and mathematical and abstract concepts. The more parents sing and/or play sacred music in the presence of their baby or young child, the more the brain generates neural circuits and patterns. It is essential then, that parents cultivate, encourage, and support their children's appreciation for music. Again, sacred music is recommended for its ability to create a high vibration and beneficial atmosphere that helps to calm children while heightening their level of intelligence and intuitive thinking. Children should be encouraged to chant along with sacred music, for this is a magical experience that forms patterns and creates energy fields of resonance and movement in the surrounding space. The energy absorbed positively alters the child's breathing, pulse, blood pressure, muscle tension, and skin temperature. Due to the high level of unfiltered noise and environmental chaos, the beneficial impact of sacred music is greater when the volume is kept low.

Spiritual music differs from mainstream music in both origin and effect. Ancient Kabbalists believed that the utterance of certain words could be used to attract luck, health and divine protection. The Rootlight Sacred Music series was created in accordance with this principle. These recordings raise one's consciousness through melody and mantra. Each contains a secret Kabbalistic formula that is in perfect harmony with the divine and creative laws of the cosmos. Therefore, each CD acts as an invisible key, opening the door to opportunities that help the individual achieve his/her innermost dreams of living a successful, fulfilling life, while smoothing the way for spiritual growth. They transform the path of misfortune, illness, and sorrow into one of abundance, health, and happiness, for these melodies and mantras have been inspired by angelic forces whose only intention is to heal mankind and inspire greatness.

True spiritual music charges your human battery, because a potent combination of angelic and planetary influences endows a specific type of Kabbalistic energy during its production. The exact nature of this energy will depend upon which spiritual benefit the experienced Kabbalist creating the musical recording wishes to bestow upon those who are listening to it or chanting along with it. Once the sacred music has been empowered with Kabbalistic energy, it acts in conjunction with the principle of universal sympathy to attract a flow of similar energy in the universe. This means that our recordings simultaneously fulfill the purpose of the cause to which they are dedicated while eradicating darkness from the life of its owner. For example, if your health is impaired, our CDs designed to assist in health related matters will act as a magnet, attracting healing energy from the universe. When you chant along with the CDs in the Rootlight Sacred Music series while using the breath in a specific manner, you connect with the universe and your deepest intuitive faculties. Your body heals, your mind settles, and your heart experiences the tranquillity of truth.

The Rootlight CDs are unparalleled in their ability to connect you, and all areas of your life, with the healing powers of the universe. They are the ultimate spiritual weapons of protection. Not only will they keep you young and healthy, they will also cut through everything that is impeding your progress on your spiritual path. These sacred CDs are necessary, transformational spiritual tools for all who want to move with grace through the turbulence that has been predicted for the years leading up to 2012, and beyond. Within each track, the spiritual sciences of Kabbalah and Kundalini-Naam yoga are woven to produce an extremely effective vehicle for the transmission of the power of the Word as it was originally intended to enlighten humankind. Moreover, these recordings were created when the moon was in a favorable position, and the heavens granted clearance for the utmost benefit for human beings. You can rely on these sacred tools to heal any aspect of your life. In difficult times, they will be your best friends. They will not let you down.

The Rootlight Sacred Music series was designed for the subconscious mind to act upon, not for intellectual understanding. All deeds are recorded in the subconscious mind. It is the subconscious mind that holds us back from becoming who we truly are, for it is the subconscious mind that has the power to block the positive and healing flow of energy from the spiritual body. Therefore, it is from the subconscious mind that we must free ourselves. Indeed, the only freedom we can consciously have is freedom from the subconscious mind and its influences. States such as depression, fear, and insecurity manifest in consciousness first. We are able to reach the highest consciousness in living when we habitually control our subconscious, refrain from relating to our seven negative karmic influences, and choose to relate to the blessed, infinite nature.

The mantras contained on Rootlight's Sacred Music series work because their powerful vibration bypasses our conscious mind (our intellect) and goes directly to our subconscious mind. There, it lodges and allows for powerful, positive, Divine suggestions to be continuously pumped into our subconscious mind. In turn, this releases the negative influences that bind us. The beauty of sacred words is that their effects linger in the subconscious mind and continue to work long after we have stopped chanting. In other words, mantra is hard at work, flushing out guilt complexes and irrational hang-ups whether we are driving, working out, at work, meditating, deeply relaxed, or asleep. They serve us for as long as it takes to clear out whatever negative thoughts, emotions, patterns, or habits are dragging us down and making us reluctant to face our Higher Self. The moment we relate to our soul, our mind becomes our servant. When the mind becomes our servant, the whole of nature automatically serves us.

As you work with the sacred music in the Rootlight series, you will begin to notice signs of change. While for some change is immediate, for most it is subtle at first. As weeks pass, the signs of change will become more noticeable. You, along with family and friends, will recognize that something has shifted and that your daily life has improved. You have gained more internal light, and it is giving your aura a glowing radiance. You have become friendlier, more lovable, and nicer to be around. You have begun to accept and love those around you, even those who used to upset you. Everyday problems appear less daunting because you are more relaxed, more at ease with the world around you, and more confident about what the future holds. This is not to say that external circumstances will suddenly become perfect. You may still encounter some trying days and situations. However, the manner in which you now approach and deal with these difficulties has been altered. With the Rootlight Sacred Music series, you have learned to manage problems that arise with grace. Our sacred music works for all, regardless of religion, race, creed or gender.

Working with the Rootlight Sacred Music series is an ongoing process during which you will gradually feel positive, desirable changes occur. These changes bring you ever closer to your inner wisdom. As your inner wisdom is strengthened and followed, the various parts of your mind come to function harmoniously so that you become a contented individual, able to move through life with greater confidence and understanding that grants the ability to accomplish goals. Over time, you will become the person you've always wanted to be, for with the release of your negative karmic influences, internal darkness moves aside so the light can shine through. It is this light that allows your heart to open fully and God to come through, directing you so that His will can be made manifest.

It takes an extraordinary combination of time, dedication, knowledge, and skill to create sacred music that will impact the soul. We believe it is the birthright of each and every person on the planet to experience the blessings invoked by these highly secret words of power once available only to the spiritual elite. Therefore, if you desire a spiritual music that possesses maximum effectiveness, we invite you to experience the

Rootlight Sacred Music series. The extraordinary quality and creative power of our sacred music speaks for itself. Those who have experienced other spiritual music and are now trying the Rootlight CDs can attest to the difference. When you add the Rootlight CDs to your library, it is akin to possessing the keys of mastery that cause the door of opportunity, once closed, to fly open. Once you embark on this spiritual journey of words and music, you will feel free to gravitate toward that which makes your soul sing.

Kabbalah and Kundalini-Naam yoga are our sacred birthright as human beings. When you work with the Divine Spiritual Wisdom, the day shall come when you will cause your immortal, incorruptible principle, lying in your spiritual body, to consume all other principles that are not allied with the eternal Truth of Life. The envelope of animal man's faculty will be stripped away so that you can appear in your original purity and splendor. Then, you will become the embodiment of the light that breathes in you. No mortal tongue can describe how bright this light is or how beautiful. Yet and still, you will perpetually live in this light, seeing it all around you and showering its brilliance onto all you encounter. Understand that the path of light is the only way to overcome the cycle of karma. Once you have mastered it, nothing can disturb you. You will live beyond the power of the cycle of time, in a healthy state of existence.

18

LUMEN DE LUMINE:
The Mantra of Mantras for Connection, Illumination, and Personal and Global Healing

LET THE MYSTICAL FIRE contained within *Lumen de Lumine*, the purifying heat of its spiritual energy, the burning heart of the Heavenly soul encapsulated in the light vibration of this sacred mantra, open your heart so you may express the infinite through your finite life. When you chant or listen to *Lumen de Lumine*, all your thoughts and actions are affected, transforming you into a spiritual sunflower turning toward the divine light of the Sun. This heavenly source acts as a magnet to draw all living matter into the realm of ultimate goodness as it simultaneously creates and regenerates all non-living matter for the perfect cosmic harmonium into which the Lord has designed all things for complete and absolute oneness in Him. *Lumen de Lumine* will open your heart, which is the center of light and the true medicine for humankind revealed by the spirit of God. It is the table the Lord laid for everyone, and the place where the true bread of the Angels is prepared. Working with the heart purifies matter by removing the pain, negative patterns, and negative veils that trap us in darkness and separate us from our true nature. When the heart is open, regeneration is possible. Regeneration signifies a detachment from impure and corruptible matter. Our immortal being is released and we can once again reclaim our beautiful, loving, original, Adamic power. This is our divine birthright. Now, more than ever, we are called upon to open our hearts. When we open our hearts, we are united with the spiritual world. The bonds of ignorance fall away as the veils of illusion are removed. As a result, we are enlightened by wisdom, guided by truth and nourished by the flames of love. Our entire being is renewed and we become the dwelling place of God. In turn, we are granted the overseership of nature, intercourse with the higher worlds, and the visible enjoyment of communion with God.

Most mantras are beneficial, as they awaken the Divine within. *Lumen de Lumine*, however, is the effective mantra of light for this time. As the mantra of all mantras, *Lumen de Lumine* will bring the mental peace that allows the path of truth to become clear. It possesses the power to open the energy centers of the body, thereby harmonizing you with the vibration of this age. When sung from the neck lock, at the point where Prana and Apana meet Sushumna, its light vibration unties the knot of ignorance. *Lumen de Lumine* is a Divine secret that uplifts humanity, and those who use it will become enlightened and become one with the Divine. Moreover, *Lumen de Lumine* is the greatest Divine key, able to unlock time and liberate you from the cycle of reincarnation safely and quickly.

Lumen de Lumine is a light equal to trillions of sun rays, as it is the light vibration from the wheel of Cosmic Energy—the Great Central Sun. It is heavenly, giving energy that is the brightest of the bright and the sweetest of the sweet. This mantra of light dispels darkness and banishes evil from one's life, as it acknowledges the Glory of the Light of the Lord. It is easy to know truth, but difficult to live it. By chanting *Lumen de Lumine*, you will experience the continual flow of light from your inner self that transforms the behavioral patterns of day to day living. Indeed, the power of *Lumen de Lumine* lies in its ability to establish a vibration between self-consciousness and Supreme consciousness that will break down all subconscious barriers. In esoteric terms, from the self to the supreme self we cross, with the power of the creator, through the cosmic flow of consciousness. Lumen de Lumine acts as a connecting bridge.

Lumen de Lumine provides a direct link to the Fountain of Light, the One Cosmic Heart. When chanting or listening to *Lumen de Lumine*, you receive assistance from the Luminous Beings who are always ready to send strength and help through the finer forces of Nature. Those who have experienced *Lumen de Lumine* understand that it is a deep vibration of Love that moves through one's being and often brings the healing tears of heaven to one's heart. *Lumen de Lumine* is the mantra that ushers in the very Light of the Universe that brings healing and nurtures our souls.

Therefore, let the nurturing power of the Divine that flows through the *Lumen de Lumine* prayer feed your energy and increase your spiritual light so that you may become a healing presence here on this earth. When you chant with this mantra, you will merge with the light of your heart. This light is the spirit of the Sun, the symbol of all that is pure, powerful, beautiful, and sublime; just as the Sun shines upon all Earth, it exists as an intelligence demonstrated as love and the impetus toward all that is good and constructive. In the context of spiritual science, light allows you to see all that has been hidden by the shadow of ignorance, for spiritual light is much more than what we think of as physical light. In our Divine Spiritual Wisdom, light refers to all beneficial entities. Once these luminous beings come to dwell within you, negative forces simply melt away.

Lumen de Lumine contains the vibration of the Christic force, the wisdom of God and the overseer of all. The Christic force is the center of the heavenly world of Light, the leader of the Community of Light. It is the essential Word through which all is created—that which was in the beginning, is now and forever shall be—and the wellspring from which light and love flow. Working with the divine sound vibrations of *Lumen de Lumine* will link you to the Community of Light. Your heart and mind will then be attuned to the energies of the divine light of this Age of the Glory of self.

The vibration of *Lumen de Lumine* describes the Glory of the Lord. Chant in the early hours before the Sun has risen, as this is the time of day when the channels to the Divine are the most clear. Your heart will open, and, in turn, charge the solar centers and connect you with the Cosmic Energy that releases you from karma. Those who chant or listen to *Lumen de Lumine* for 11 minutes a day while meditating on the light of the Sun will overcome all challenges and rule their destiny.

Rose Croix Kabbalists chant *Lumen de Lumine* in order to remove darkness. When used consciously, this mantra provides a potent shield of protection and healing, as you are establishing a spiritual communion with the hierarchy of Luminous Beings who dwell in the invisible world, as well as calling on the help and protection of the hosts of the superior astral world. All you need to contribute is sincerity, reverence and humility.

In other words, chanting or listening to *Lumen de Lumine* will create a communion between you and the beneficent and benevolent hosts of the superior astral world. It is the mantra of physical protection against the ill will of other people. It is a prayer of the strongest potency which will keep misfortune away and bring peace, love and mercy in the lives of those who chant or listen to it.

If you are faced with challenges, play *Lumen de Lumine* continuously and it will eat the darkness out of your life. By offering a *Lumen de Lumine* to a loved one, you are giving them the highest gift, which is light. Give light as a present and God will bless you ten times in various ways. Just listen to it and it will purify and strengthen your aura. Play it in a room and it will clear the energy in a short time. Go to sleep with it; you will wake up vitalized. We recommend that you listen to and/or chant this mantra in order to create communion between you and the luminous beings.

As you work with *Lumen de Lumine* each morning, keep your mind focused on the Sun so that you connect mentally with its vivifying power. *Lumen de Lumine* holds the power of the Sun's rays, and is a symbol of the ineffable presence of the supreme principle. It brings light and illumination, energy and strength, hope and love. As you listen to the heavenly energy of *Lumen de Lumine*, it holds your entire being within its healing and soothing vibrations. While working with this sacred sound, imagine that you are storing the Sun's healing rays in the cells of your brain, particularly in your solar plexus, which acts like a reservoir of energies from which you can draw light in order to accomplish your daily tasks. This will recharge you so that you are able to greet the day tirelessly with beauty, bounty, and bliss. Those who listen to *Lumen de Lumine* are surrounded by an aura of shimmering sunlight, and it brings the presence of the luminous beings at their four sides. With *Lumen de Lumine* you create a communion between yourself and the beneficent, benevolent hosts of the higher worlds. This will warm your heart, and give you the feeling of joy, security, and safety that releases your soul from the trap of darkness.

In the end, all creatures resemble their environment. When you spend time listening to or chanting along with *Lumen de Lumine* while simultaneously contemplating the Sun and soaking up its light with your being, you will become like the Sun. Therefore, use this heavenly sound current and adopt the Sun as your model. You will watch yourself becoming luminous, warmhearted, and vibrant with life. Those who meditate on *Lumen de Lumine* and the Sun will find themselves blessed each day with many rewards.

Let the projection of your psyche be nothing but light; let each person who meets you be healed and uplifted by the strength and beauty of that light. Concentrate on the light of the Sun and immerse yourself in the energy of *Lumen de Lumine*. You will experience the radiance of your heart center, and expand beyond the limits of time and space into the realm of total peace and joy that allows you to know your boundlessness.

Meditation for Bringing in Light

PREPARATION

Put your hands on the heart center to create a neutrality of the magnetic field. Close your eyes. Breathe deeply. With each inhale, welcome the breath, and with each exhale send all sickness out of the body. The longer and deeper you breathe, the more you will start to feel lighter, brighter and beautiful. Slow and deep breathing automatically controls the mind and causes the motor system in the brain to readjust the entire function of the body so that it is under your physical control. Once things come under your physical control, your positive, hidden subconscious desires, such as being healthy, strong and prosperous, are given a chance to manifest. As your heartfelt prayers begin to project out of you, the body creates the environment needed to crystallize them.

TIME: 3-11 minutes. To end, inhale very deeply, exhale. Inhale deeply, expand your shoulders as well as your chest and exhale. Inhale very deeply, expand your body and relax.

Recommended music: *Sounds of the Ether* CD, track 5

PART I: Lumen de Lumine

Sit in easy pose place the hands, palms facing up, in front of the diaphragm, with the left wrist underneath the right. In other words the back of the right wrist is resting on top of the left rascettes.* With your hands in this posture, eyes closed, listen to or chant along with the *Lumen de Lumine* CD for 3-11 minutes. To end, inhale very deeply, exhale. Inhale deeply, expand your shoulders as well as your chest and exhale. Inhale very deeply, expand your body and relax.

Lumen de Lumine
Deum de Deo
Lumen de Lumine
Deum Verum de Deo Vero
Lumen de Lumine

* The three lines that generally run parallel to one another on the wrist and mark the lower boundary of the palm are referred to as the bracelets of life. These lines, represent the longevity and the state of health of a person. They also stand the past, present and future. Each line corresponds to approximately 26-30 years of life. When taken together, they are called the rascettes. Generally speaking, these three lines indicate the weaknesses or strengths of the body's internal organs, specifically in relation to childbirth. The first of these lines, closest to the palm, is often called the Venus bracelet. It is the most important in determining how many children are likely to be born, and is especially significant when it rises in the form of an arch. When looking at this line, Kabbalah and yoga masters very special cases forbade the subject to have children, as it was a sign of unusual suffering in childbirth. Often, dangers to the mother's life during delivery are indicated. The Venus bracelet also shows whether one will have a large family or not. When the second line acts the same way, it supports the first. Three good lines can indicate strong health.

PART II: I Am That I Am

Sit in any comfortable meditative position. With your upper arms close to your sides, bring your hands side by side to the level of your heart and cupped as if you were receiving something. Eyes are closed. Listen to or chant along with track 2 on the *Sounds of the Ether* CD. Know that you are blessed and allow all the blessings of heaven to flow to you. As you feel the boundless flow of spirit, ask for whatever you need. There is no minimum or maximum time for this meditation.

I Am I Am helps you to realize that you are a point of light within God's mind, and a point of love within the Lord's heart. Each one of us must realize that we are indeed made in God's image and likeness. We are One and nothing can separate us. Know that one aspect of God is, God can be and God cannot be. This means that God in the world is finite and infinite. But those who have found God within God are the infinity in its own orbit. They look like humans: they possess flesh and bones, with faces and extremities. Yet, they speak in a healing manner, invoking the greatness that lives within us. People follow them. Everything in their existence is uplifting, healing and balanced. And beyond this existence, they have the one thing which money cannot buy and nothing can sell, upon which no value can be placed. For these beings live in God consciousness, which is the everlasting infinity of grace. This is priceless. Whosoever works with our Divine Spiritual Wisdom accepts the high consciousness, the will of God, and becomes God within himself or herself. Let the power of the Spirit of God flow in and through you. As you listen to or chant along with I Am I Am. Open yourself up to this infinite power.

Lumen de Lumine and *I Am I Am* will cause you to walk towards God. As you take one step towards the Divine, the Divine shall walk 1,000 steps towards you.

PART III: Recite the Prayer of Love, Peace and Light

Love before me	*Peace before me*	*Light before me*
Love behind me	*Peace behind me*	*Light behind me*
Love at my left	*Peace at my left*	*Light at my left*
Love at my right	*Peace at my right*	*Light at my right*
Love above me	*Peace above me*	*Light above me*
Love below me	*Peace below me*	*Light below me*
Love in me	*Peace in me*	*Light in me*
Love in my surroundings	*Peace in my surroundings*	*Light in my surroundings*
Love to all	*Peace to all*	*Light to all*
Love to the universe	*Peace to the universe*	*Light to the universe*

PART IV: Long Deep Breathing

Put your hands on the heart center to create a neutrality of the magnetic field. Breathe deeply and mechanically to automatically calm the mind. Welcome the breath in and affectionately send it out with all the sickness and tensions of the body. Breathe deeply and mechanically to automatically control the mind. The longer and deeper you breathe, the more you will start changing, you will start feeling lighter, brighter and beautiful. The eyes remain closed.

TIME: Continue for 11 minutes. To end, inhale very deeply, exhale. Inhale deeply, expand your shoulders as well as your chest and exhale. Inhale very deeply, expand your body and relax.

19

ACHIEVING COSMIC CONSCIOUSNESS

Whoever vibrates the holy Naam of God is and shall be liberated, for wherever Naam is heard the ear is ravished, the mind is cleaned and the mouth is filled with a pleasant savor. The mere utterance of Naam removes negativity and scatters temptation. Naam strengthens the heart, healing all conflicts between the world and the flesh. It is the force that causes darkness to flee, cures illnesses and awakens the soul with every heavenly delight. Whoever vibrates Naam, then, shall see their enemies reduced to nothingness and shall flourish in health, happiness and the abundance of peace. The Creator, that Great Architect of the Universe, does wondrous things for those who vibrate Naam. Blessed be his glorious Name. The power of Naam shall endure as long as the bright Sun and beyond, shining its blessing upon the earth and mankind forever. Mighty miracles are performed by the sole power of the most precious vibration of Naam.

Sacred Naam is the giver of life; the sacred name of salvation and joy. It is the Prana, the Pavan Guru. Naam is the undying spirit of God. It is a most divine computerized combination designed to stimulate your higher consciousness and shield you from the pain of life. Reciting Naam will remove your fear, and give you internal strength and a solid feeling of infinity, for it will give you the totality of Godhood. It will grant you the strength to bring in Love, Peace and Light. Understand that the Divine Spiritual Wisdom is the most positive, healing system. Through vibrating Naam, you can always clean your spirit, and obtain purity and piety so that you may experience the reality of Love. Vibrate the Naam and the Universe shall serve you. Vibrate the Naam and let the whole earth be filled with the glory of God.

In order to understand this life, you must understand that Naam is a gift from God and the life line that will save you during this Dark Age, also known as *Kali Yug*. Let's examine what Kali Yug means. One year in the life of the sun is equivalent to 360 human years and forms the unit of a divine year. One day of *Brahma* is equivalent to 12,000 divine years and 4,320,000 human years. This period is called a *Kalpa*. A Kalpa, or one day of Brahma, divides into four Ages. The first is *Sat Yug* with a length of 1,728,000 human years; the second is *Treta Yug* with a length of 1,296,000 human years; the third is *Doapar Yug* with a length of 864,000 human years; and the fourth is *Kali Yug* with a length of 432,000 human years. The ratio created by the length of these ages is 4:3:2:1. Interestingly, this ratio is found in many sacred computations. Now, taken together, the four Yugs make 4,320,000 Earth years, called the *Maha Yug*, or Great Ages.

The scriptures describe the four Ages of the Maha Yug. Sat Yug was the Age of Truth, or the Golden Age when Truth reigned supreme. During this Age, man was one with the Divine. He realized the vibration that this Cosmic Energy created to make *Prakriti* (manifestation). During this era, man meditated on the Naam, ONG—the vibration of the Divine. Treta Yug was the Silver Age when Truth was three-quarters revealed. Treta Yug was a period of sacrificial oblations. During this Age, man was weakened and he recited the Naam, *Sohang*. Sohang acknowledged his identity with the Divine, which means "I am thou." Doapar Yug was the Age of half-veiled Truth when idol worship was law. During this Age, man recited, *Ong Namo Narayana*. Kali Yug, the fourth Age in which we find ourselves, is called the Dark Age or Age of Iron and Steel. Here, in the Age of the Machine that is represented by another wheel that runs it, the Truth is three quarters veiled. Constant vibrations from that wheel of Cosmic energy give power of life movement to this wheel of creation. When you draw one circle like the wheel and put another circle like a wheel over it (wheel over wheel), you get the figure 8, which, according to the science of Numerology, represents Infinity turned sideways. Each one of the four great Ages is followed by great changes in the configuration of the planetary continents. This is why our current Age is experiencing such upheaval and profound change. With Truth veiled so significantly during the Dark Age, we need a potent tool to lift the veil.

The particular Naam on *The Seal of Higher Destiny* CD is the master key of this Age. Understand that the energy of Naam permeates and pervades throughout all of the Rootlight CDs. Those who rise in the ambrosial hours and vibrate Naam will cause the heavens to protect them, heal them, and take care of every area of their life. Indeed, Naam is the most potent and supreme remedy of this age of the glory of Self. It is vital to healing and liberation.

The power of Naam has been acknowledged as the direct and true way from Ancient Egypt and the pharaoh, Akhaneton or Ikhnaton, who ruled from 1379 to 1362 BC, to St. John the Baptist and Christ, to the ten Sikh Gurus, beginning with Guru Nanak. In keeping with this tradition, the sound current will be the highest principle of this Age. All other spiritual practices will soon bow to the way of Naam, as Naam Yoga is the custodian of the powers of the rays of the sun, and is aligned with the healing, beneficial laws of the Cosmic. It is the bringer of love, faith, and hope, of light and enlightenment, of energy and strength. Naam is the shield of protection and the guardian of the weak and innocent. Naam is the essence of this world, and the Custodian and Guardian of Kundalini Shakti. Naam is the giver of life to the living, the giver of joy to the sorrowful, and the bringer of compassion to the lost and lonely. As human vice peaks during this Age, and we are subject to all manner of earthly and physical disturbances, practice Naam so that your eyes may be opened and your protective shields strengthened. It will cause you to stand eternally in the light, guided and guarded by the luminous beings. Through Universal Kabbalah, Naam will reveal the mysteries of your life, as well as the duties and destinies you carried with you into this incarnation. In turn, you will be able to reach out and receive love, light and healing, as you embrace the true destiny of your spiritual path and begin the work that you have been prepared to do. As soon as you start practicing Naam, you will feel the presence of the luminous beings with you at all times. They are there to provide you with guidance, love, and strength. The Sikh scriptures testify in plain words that during the four Grand Divisions of time people benefited from the practice of Naam by sitting at the feet of those who have become the Word made flesh. Naam alone will be the saving Light of this Age and beyond.

Working with the Naam on *The Seal of Higher Destiny* will bring the radiance of the Sun into your heart and the vastness of the universe into your soul. The yoga of Naam is the highest method of contact with God, which causes the soul to engage in a beautiful union with spirit as it attains indescribable bliss. It projects the mind beyond the realm of everyday, earthly consciousness into the infinity of the cosmos, thereby increasing your sense of personal relatedness to the infinite identity. The after effect of vibrating Naam brings the utmost peace, bliss, and joy. By mastering this Naam you gain vision of the higher world and perceive the endless manifestation of the light of God. The universe has been created by the Divine will. When you attune yourself to it through this Naam, there will come a point where the things that you need will simply come to you by willing. This Naam grants understanding of the greatness of He who spoke and brought the Universe into being, while eradicating your individual karma. Communing with God in this manner will clean your mind, comfort your heart, heal your body, and enliven your spirit. The easiest way to overcome disease, disappointments, and disasters is to be in constant attunement with God, for the supreme help comes from attuning with the spirit.

Eck Ong Kar Sat Nam Siri Wahe Guru is a Naam that causes you to tread the road of wisdom safely. It causes you to enter cosmic consciousness and commune with God. If you desire to stop the cycle of time and be liberated from the loop of life and death, this is the Naam for you. *Eck Ong Kar Sat Nam Siri Wahe Guru* means: *There is One God whose name is truth, highest wondrous One who brings light.* It will bring you closer to freedom from karma and the cycle of reincarnation. Baba Siri Chand, a renowned mystic and figure of tremendous spiritual power, used the above Naam. Born in 1494, Baba Siri Chand was the eldest son of Guru Nanak, the first Sikh Guru. As a child, he displayed a contemplative nature, which inspired Guru Nanak to prescribe a life of an Udasi for him. Baba Siri Chand persistently sat in samadhi with the name of God. Because of his disciplined and dedicated meditation, the great bounty of God's gifts flowed through him. Indeed, an ocean of God's blessings poured forth from his merciful gaze. Indians of all religions flocked to see him, becoming followers who not only loved him, but also prayed to him. By practicing and imbibing his father's teachings, Baba Siri Chand became a respected leader in his own right. A survey conducted during the reign of the Emperor Jehangir found that Baba Siri Chand was the most influential saint in India. When the Emperor asked Mian Mir, his own darvesh (a powerful, truthful, God-intoxicated holy person) who the greatest darvesh was, Mian Mir replied, "At this time the elder son of Guru Nanak is king of the darveshes." In truth, Baba Siri Chand was not only revered by the average people of all sects and religions, but also, he was highly respected by yogis, saints, kings, and the Sikh Gurus. The first six Sikh Gurus sought and revered his guidance, many of whom offered their sons to him in service. However, even though his life was a continuous miracle, Baba Siri Chand never called attention to himself. Rather, he and his followers, known as Udasis, spread the message of his father in a nonsectarian and universalist manner, that emphasized meditation on God's Holy Name, hard work, and service to those in need. At the great age of 149, after finishing a lecture, Baba Siri Chand stood up and said, "I am leaving now." The year was 1643, and he left the visible world with his body intact. He simply walked away dressed as he was and wearing sandals. Stepping onto a rock in a rushing river, Baba Siri Chand was carried safely across. He was beyond the cycle of life and death, for he is one with the eternal light of God, one with that eternal Power of which all the scriptures have spoken. Even though he lived in the world, he remained beyond the world. He has existed for thousands of years now, and even though we cannot see him with our external eyes, he is still with us.

Rootlight's twelfth CD, *The Seal of Higher Destiny*, which contains the Naam *Eck Ong Kar Sat Nam Siri Wahe Guru*, was inspired by a spiritual and mysterious encounter I had in India. Before I describe this unusual meeting, I need to say that as I traveled along my spiritual path, I have experienced many spiritual encounters on various continents. Also, since childhood, I had and continue to have encounters in the invisible world with the various luminous beings that dwell therein, where they instruct me and inspire my actions. I am grateful for these encounters to the depth of my soul, for they have provided constant guidance and protection in the achievement of the Great Work.

Humans stand at the dawn of 2012, and feel inside their heart the grip of change, the twists and turns of destiny that lie within their grasp that beckon and tempt them to follow. And now, more than ever, humankind needs all the help it can get in order to evolve into men and women of light. Therefore, human beings are adjusting and attuning to the evolution of the planet, which is allowing them to acclimate to the radiance of the light of the new Age. There are currently many active, visible and invisible agents of light trying to help save the earth from self-destruction. Some are helping from the unseen world, while others are acting in the visible realm. Of these, some are silently completing the work backstage, while others are front and center. It makes no difference, for the masters all come from the same source of light. Most of their work is largely done in silence, in order to contribute to the existence and order of the universe, assisting the Divine in fulfillment of its plan for evolution and expansion. They not only appear on all continents, but also, they are working together in synchronicity. The teachings I present derive from the One Source, the One Truth, the One Sun. They are the teachings of the wise who have gone before, who have walked the earth many times, in many forms, during many ages, and wearing many faces. Through the cycle of incarnation, they have transcended the need to continue their evolution in the limited reality in which we find ourselves. They now reside in the invisible realm of light. It is via these sacred teachings that they seek to guide humankind to the next level of being. It is up to you to do your part in transforming the earth by raising your own vibration and expanding your level of consciousness. Men and women need to awaken to the cosmic truths.

In regard to a profound spiritual encounter, I had begun my trip in Israel in December 2004, but I felt myself being pulled to India, a country I had visited six months earlier. Consequently, at the end of my stay in Israel, I flew to India. When I arrived, I had the most incredible experience. A tall and beautiful holy man with a long and snowy white beard, Maharaj Ji, appeared to me in a dream state. He not only confirmed the veracity of the power of the Word as a pure way of binding with God, but he also gave me additional means through which I could employ an infinitude of healing applications for the betterment of humankind. Exactly three days later, shortly after 11:00pm on the 25th of December—a day devoted to the worship of Christ Consciousness—I met Maharaj Ji in person. He appeared as he had appeared in my dream state, with a pure, radiant, vast aura. Speaking with enormous love, goodness, and affection, he said that he had come to me in my dreams. He was surrounded by people who were graceful, kind, and very serviceful. What occurred during my encounter with this holy man is beyond words. You may be able to grasp more of the great significance of this encounter when I tell you that Baba Siri Chand, king of the darveshes, and known to have tremendous spiritual power, has been instructing Maharaj Ji since childhood. To this day, these two amazing beings are in celestial communication. I received many, many blessings during this divinely orchestrated encounter, and between the time of our meeting and my subsequent departure, incredible things happened. I need to add here that it was during this meeting that the Maharaj Ji had bestowed upon me a version of *Eck Ong Kar Sat Nam Siri Wahe Guru* with fueled power.

The raw form of *The Seal of Higher Destiny* was first introduced during one of my New Year's classes. It attuned a room full of one hundred men and women from all walks of life to the heavens, raising their consciousness to such a degree that all experienced an indescribable spiritual high. The rate of vibration created was powerfully healing. Time flew by, and those in attendance left wanting more. When mantra is practiced in a group under the direction of someone with extensive practice and reverence for the power of the Word, the psychic and inner unfolding of everyone in the group is greatly enhanced. This is due to the fact that an atmosphere of higher etheric vibration is created in the environment; when 100 people chant a perfect permutation and combination of sacred words such as those on the Rootlight CDs, and they are heard by the same 100 people, the power of the vibration is squared, causing a vibrational healing impact of 10,000 in strength on the psyche of each person present. The concentrated and highly charged vibrations of such a harmonious group attract heavenly vibrations of great potency, resulting in an increased stimulation of all spiritual faculties. The New York Wednesday night class at Universal Force Healing Center gives similar benefits.

It is important to recognize that as you learn the Divine Spiritual Wisdom and practice the sacred words revealed on the Rootlight Sacred Music series, you will generate a healing energy that extends for a 25-mile radius. (The radius extends even further for those who possess high levels of consciousness, such as masters. This explains why the work of one highly evolved being can benefit an entire city, or sometimes a country.) If you desire to bind your soul to the higher world, meditate along with the mantra on *The Seal of Higher Destiny*. Not only will you be liberated, but no evil shall befall you, because God's name will be with you constantly. As with the other Rootlight CDs, the principles of Universal Kabbalah have been perfectly woven into its production. (This is especially true of the second track.) While the form of the Naam recorded on the first track is well known among those who practice Kundalini yoga, the second track was directly inspired by my divine encounter in India. This mantra takes care of the tenth gate, the gate of salvation. It is at the top of the head (fontanel), and the pineal gland is located underneath it. It hardens as the child grows older.

This mantra causes the pineal and pituitary glands to enter into a beneficial, vibratory relationship. The pineal secretes, and the pituitary becomes the radar that detects negativity and keeps your mind away from it. It awakens your soul. When your soul is awakened, everything begins to work for you automatically. Your intuitive and psychic powers are activated. You are able to look into the future and, in so doing, are able to align yourself with the energies that contribute to the existence and order of the universe, and assist the Divine in fulfillment of Its plan for evolution and expansion. You become opened to God's light, and filled with the Divine wisdom that lies within the human heart. As this Divine wisdom becomes the driving force in your life, you come to know the totality of your surroundings. You become a blessed being, actively engaged in an evolutionary process of knowing that ultimately leads to peace and harmony. This mantra will help you find God in your heart. You will begin to hunger for the sweet wine of this beautiful Divine Spiritual Wisdom, for reconnecting with your higher self is the ultimate catalyst for all development, harmony, and spiritual growth.

This Naam takes one to *Aad*. *Aad* means the beginning. The beginning which is infinity. It has the power to open all the energy centers in your body and to harmonize you with the vibration of this age. This mantra is the light that dispels darkness. When chanted, no darkness or negativity can stand against it. Practice with this mantra, so that, in the essence of your nucleus and the nucleus of your essence, you may activate the interior organ of your spiritual body. As a result, it allows you to emanate life in such a way that it reveals everything to you and opens all the doors to you. It opens your inner eyes and ears, and you begin to see the invisible realities. Blessed are those who practice with this Naam and make the High One their trust. For goodness and kindness shall follow them all the days of their life.

Whosoever in this Machine Age will meditate and recite this Naam, which praises the Lord and has eight vibrations, will open the lock of ignorance and darkness and this will liberate the being and unite him with the Divine. *Eck Ong Kar Sat Nam Siri Wahe Guru* has eight vibrations and describes the Glory of the Lord.

Thus said the Master, "In the time period 2 1/2 hours before the rising of the sun when the channels are most clear, if the mantra is sung in sweet harmony, you will be one with the Lord." This will open the solar plexus, which in turn will charge the solar center—they will get connected with the Cosmic Energy and thus man will be liberated from the time cycle of karma.

The long *Eck Ong Kar* mantra enables us to avoid all unnecessary troubles of life. It gives all knowledge which has ever existed in the universe of universes, and opens the third eye, the command center.

When you vibrate with this Naam, the whole world resounds with you. This is pure ecstasy. With this mantra your mental frequency becomes "there is One who is All and I am a small part of that All." As soon as you realize this truth, the things you need come to you. It will make you expand, and all will be done for you by the universe.

You will simply become sovereign. This Naam causes your pranic flow to mix with your psyche and joins Prakirti, the natural flow, and life becomes very serviceful.

It causes you to master yourself. As you master yourself, God loves you, and His mastery shines through the various levels of your being. As a result, you become healthy, happy and joyful. Use the Naam and let heaven pluck you from the net that has been laid secretly by negative forces. Those who master this Naam shall inherit the land of light and delight in the abundance of peace, love and joy. This mantra praises God who is the King of the Earth. This Naam causes heaven to purify you, to wash you with light so that you may be whiter than snow. It grants you a pure heart, renews you with the right spirit and restores you with the joy of a liberated soul. This Naam opens up the *Trikutee, kamal bigaasai*. It gives one the experience of ecstasy by opening the inner center of the brain.

Meditation to Awaken Your Highest Destiny

POSITION:
Sit straight in a cross-legged position. Eyes are closed.

MANTRA: **Eck Ong Kaar – Sat Naam Siree – Wa-he Guru**
Chant from the navel in a two and one-half breath cycle.

TIME:
Continue for 11 minutes. To end, inhale deeply, hold the breath tight, and squeeze every fiber of your body. Exhale. Repeat two more times. Relax.

COMMENTS:
Each sound vibrates and integrates a different chakra within the aura. Take a deep inhale and chant *Eck Ong Kar*. *Eck* is very short, as when we split the atom, releasing a humongous amount of energy from the first chakra. *Ong* is vibrated from the second chakra, resonating through the nostrils to experience the conch of the third eye. *Kar* is vibrated from the navel. Take another deep inhale and chant *Sat Naam Siree*. *Sat* is short, coming abruptly from the navel, pulling up the diaphragm. *Naam* is very long and resonates through the heart. *Siree*, the greatest of all the great powers, the Shakti—is chanted with the last bit of breath. It is pulled from the navel and up through the neck lock. Then take a short half breath and chant *Wah-hey Guroo*. *Wahe* and *Guru* are released through the top of the head.

Through this meditation you will master the power of prana, *Pavan Siddhi*—until the breath of life becomes your own. It will give you *Vac Siddhi*—the power of speech. What you say with the breath shall happen. It is hard labor. Do this Jaap, repeating it again and again, until you reach 1/10 of the day—2 1/2 hours. Your face will be bright and beautiful, and you will settle the accounts of everyone you know.

*Good health is the result of perfect rhythm and tone.
When our physical health is not functioning
at an optimum level, it means that
the music of our body is out of sync.
Harmony and rhythm of music is necessary
to bring the body into a similar state of
harmony and rhythm.*

*Sacred music is a productive healing tool
precisely because it is comprised of
rhythm, tone, and harmony.*

20

THE HEALING SPIRIT OF RA MA DA SA

To initiate self-healing and for protection against all known and unknown diseases, work with the *Ra Ma Da Sa* mantra. The simple yet timeless truth of *Ra Ma Da Sa* allows you to gracefully face health challenges as you move through time and space. *Ra Ma Da Sa* is a concentrated form of spiritual healing used by Master yogis for thousands of years to build bodily resistance to disease and treat a myriad of ailments. In fact, they believed *Ra Ma Da Sa* acted as an energetic tonic, improving the circulation and flow of prana throughout the entire body. This completely beneficial mantra strengthens the energy field and improves every aspect of your life. Chanting it automatically transforms the negative into positive, effectively revitalizing the body. The health benefits of this healing mantra just cannot be ignored. When you listen to or chant *Ra Ma Da Sa*, disease, pain and sorrow move out of your life, granting you liberation from disease and freedom to move toward greater happiness.

When you listen to *Ra Ma Da Sa*, focusing on the words and tune while sitting down, you instantly feel the power of life and the light of heaven that dispels all internal darkness in your heart. *Ra Ma Da Sa* is the perfect healing formula, the source of new life that grants the practitioner complete and total cellular rebirth in 120 days. In a manner that is beyond words, this mantra fortifies the immune system in ways that are unmatched by both medicinal herbs and modern drugs alike. Your breath is a potent tool here. When you chant along with the *Ra Ma Da*

Sa CD, the power of your breath becomes so balanced, so purified and developed that it attracts all the healing elements you could get from herbs, flowers, fruits, and other natural remedies. You can attain as much healing as you desire if you work with *Ra Ma Da Sa*. Its capacity to serve is infinite. Simply by being in the presence of its healing vibrations, you will receive its benefits automatically. *Ra Ma Da Sa* is so powerful that it will bring you health and peace even if they are not written in the stars for you. It will even heal those who cannot pronounce the words correctly.

After almost thirty years of teaching, healing, and working with thousands of individuals of every race, gender, religion, and class, I realized that I needed to choose a universal and elegant mantra especially for those plagued with health problems. In order to do so, I needed to find a sacred sound that would work for anyone, in any situation, in any country, without the limitations that constant ritual and overly formalized structures often place on those who are physically restricted with ill health. Indeed, when I first began reaching out to those with acute health and spiritual challenges, finding the most efficient and effective way to help and heal proved challenging at times. Each person and situation required that I sift through the most vital and important of the sacred teachings, and then make them accessible and compatible with the religious beliefs, cultural customs, and individual challenge of the person before me so that they could receive immediate help.

In my restless desire to find a solution for my students, friends, and clients, I began to petition the cosmic for guidance. This is how *Ra Ma Da Sa Sa Say So Hung*, in the form that it appears on the Rootlight CD was revealed to me. I can confidently say that *Ra Ma Da Sa* is one of the most powerful mantras known and is extraordinarily effective in dealing with health challenges. It is powerful. It is universal. It works on all levels—mental, spiritual, emotional, and physical.

Ra Ma Da Sa Sa Say So Hung is called the *Shushmana Mantra*. It contains the eight sounds that stimulate the Kundalini to flow in the central channel of the spine and in the spiritual centers. This sound balances the five zones of the left and right hemispheres of the brain in order to activate the neutral mind. As this happens, the hypothalamus pulsates in rhythm with the divine gland, causing the pituitary master gland to tune the entire glandular system. Then the sympathetic, parasympathetic, and active nervous systems match the timing of the glandular system. As a result, the muscular system and cells in the blood work in conjunction to receive the healing vibration, triggering the process of rebuilding one's health.

Ra Ma Da Sa is a rare diamond that connects you with the pure healing energy of the universe. In addition to working on the body's physical systems, this mantra can purify the aura and consolidate your mental projection into a one-pointed positivity directed towards yourself and your health. Listening to it helps rebalance the entire auric circulation and gives you a sense of security that activates your self-healing capacities. A consistent listening or chanting practice becomes impressive enough to permeate the subconscious, which in turn automatically influences the conscious mind. When this occurs, the mantra becomes a part of your deep, intuitional conviction. In other words, you can instill the health trend in your consciousness by injecting this strong healing vibration into your mind. Your actions and whole being will then obey that thought. In order to change health troubles, we must alter the process of thought that brings the crystallization of consciousness into different forms of matter and action. This recording, which is set to a healing classical tune, helps you develop the pattern of health.

Each hour of the day is under the influence of a planet and the luminous beings inhabiting that planet. Therefore, each hour that comes and goes brings entities that work on minerals, plants, animals, and human beings. Moreover, each planet is aligned with specific colors and sounds. The symphony of sounds, then, varies with each hour of the day according to each succession of spirit. As the planets sing in space, the whole universe sings, immersing us in its beautiful music and the music of the spheres. Animated by the hymns of the angels, the universe breathes and nourishes itself. It is through prayer and contemplation that we can perceive the symphony of the planets to which the angelic hierarchies are linked. Understand that the spiritual plane is structured and organized in such a way that certain sacred mantras can lead you exactly where you want to be. Chanting or listening to the Rootlight *Ra Ma Da Sa* CD delivers you to the region of health. In other words, when you work with

Rootlight's *Ra Ma Da Sa* CD you visit the realms of the invisible world where the gift of health is found and obtained.

Good health is the result of perfect rhythm and tone. When our physical health is not functioning at an optimum level, it means that the music of our body is out of sync. In this instance, the harmony and rhythm of music is necessary to bring the body into a similar state of harmony and rhythm. Sacred music is a productive healing tool precisely because it is comprised of rhythm, tone, and harmony. *Ra Ma Da Sa* provides the exact healing rhythm and words needed by those experiencing health problems. The mantra and the classical tune we have set to it, with its ideal tone and rhythm, is a perfectly structured healing code that gives nourishment to those who hear it by creating the vibration necessary for good health in the body. Those who then chant along with it are granted even greater levels of healing, health, and longevity.

Scientific research attests to the developmental benefits of classical music on children. Classical music seems to impart balance, and most scientists believe there is something special about its structure that makes the brain respond positively. After birth, a child's brain continues to develop. Therefore, it is possible to heighten both a child's prenatal and postnatal intelligence. The most powerful period of brain development—a critical window of opportunity—starts at birth and ends around the age of 11. Recent studies have shown that the neurological foundations for problem-solving and general reasoning are largely established by age one. The spoken language an infant hears creates a complex set of interconnections, which has an important impact on overall brain development. Similarly, studies suggest that the more parents sing or play melodious and structured music to their baby, the more the baby's brain generates neural circuits and patterns.

Scientific research now also suggests that the adult brain responds to music almost as if it were medicine. Hans Jenny, a Swiss engineer and doctor, describes the science of how sound and vibration interact with matter. Vibrating sounds form patterns and create energy fields of resonance and movement in the surrounding space. As we absorb these energies, they subtly alter our breathing, pulse, blood pressure, muscle tension, skin temperature, and other internal rhythms. It comes as no surprise that clinical studies and the anecdotal evidence of music therapists suggest that music can be employed to manage pain, moods, depression, blood pressure, and anxiety, as well as the nausea associated with chemotherapy and the immobility associated with Parkinson's disease. Specifically, a study from Stanford University School of Medicine showed a significant reduction in depression in 20 people ranging in age from 61 to 86 who listened to familiar music while practicing various stress-reduction techniques. During the eight-week trial period, the control group, who were not exposed to music or therapeutic exercise, showed no improvement. Music has also been shown to lessen the need for sedatives and pain relievers during and after surgery. Many medical practitioners, believing that music can play an instrumental role in lessening a patient's post-surgery recovery time and help them to better cope with future complications, now recommend that music be incorporated into traditional healing modalities. Sacred music, in particular, can help patients as it creates a positive, uplifting environment, and enables them to better deal with what they are going through.

Having discussed benefits of *Ra Ma Da Sa*, as well as the scientific support of the use of music and sacred sounds as healing tools, let's turn our attention to the specific structure of the *Ra Ma Da Sa* mantra. A diseased state can be symbolically called the death of Christ. When we are struck with disease, it is like passing into the shadow of death as the Sun of our being descends during the crucifixion that is disease. This occurs when Saturn, the lord of Karma governed by the number 8, is present. Eight is significant, as it is the number of infinity. The longest chapter of the Bible, Psalm 119, is divided into 22 sections, which are then divided into eight verses. The fact that *Ra Ma Da Sa* is segmented into eight sounds demonstrates the hand of God at work. Indeed, the structure of the *Ra Ma Da Sa* mantra presents in itself such a number of remarkable coincidences that one is forced to conclude that the position of the eight healing sounds were purposely planned to come together for a definite reason. The relationship of such a coincidence will sooner or later strike the seeker of truth as an illustration of divine design, and consequently, proof of the divine inspiration that guided the masters and yogis who handed it down.

A look at how this healing mantra contributes to the overall health of a person is very fascinating. The virtues of this healing mantra seem to extend itself beyond normal peripheries. Every sound seems to play an important role. The sounds of *Ra Ma Da Sa Sa Say So Hung* are so significant in their spiritual meaning that they reveal and epitomize the great healing truth of the ages. *RA* is the basis of all life. It is the fire principle that represents the Sun, which is the first cause, the creator, and the visible symbol of God. Were it not for the Sun showering us with the pranic life force, life would not exist on Earth. Because it is both the beginning and that by which everything is created, it represents all that is creative, positive, and healing. It is the simplest essence of divinity, the root of all things, a center of spiritual energy that is full of endless life, activity, and force.

Kabbalistically speaking, the Sun is a projection of the first sphere of the Tree of Life, Kether, with its first name of God, Eheieh, the name of the divine essence. The Sun's symbolic number is one, the first of the ten digits that represents the manifold expression of deity, conceived of as the creative power of the primal light. The Sun can be symbolically associated with *Raysheeth ha gigoleem*, the first whirlings or impulse, and represents a concentration of light energy within the infinity of Ain Soph which sets in motion the process of being revealed. All beginnings, all seeds, all things come from the Sun, this sphere of the energy of "I Am that I Am." The Sun, then, is the door through which God acts on everything, because the Sun is the heart of our universe, working with it is the highest practice of Kabbalah. By chanting or listening to *Ra Ma Da Sa*, we cause the powerful healing light of the Sun to move from the shadows of the night as our personal Christ. The Sun of righteousness rises from our symbolic tomb to restore health.

MA, the water principle, is the energy of the Moon. It is cooling and nurturing. Ma calls on the cosmos through the sound of compassion. It renders the universe the mother and you the child, a relationship that brings you help and healing.

The sounds *RA* and *MA* stimulate strength and vitality by replenishing the body's positive and negative energies. They should be intoned when you feel that your energy has been depleted. Masculine in nature,

RA represents power and authority, and depicts the positive polarity and force in the universe. Feminine in nature, *MA* is the nurturing, protective mother force in the universe represented by the negative, passive polarity of cosmic forces. Together, they stimulate physical energy and health, while strengthening one's magnetic quality and its accompanying vital aura. The presence of *RA MA*, as the bringer of life, at the beginning of this healing mantra follows the healing law of the mysterious and wonderful design involved in its construction.

DA, the Earth principle, provides the ground for action. *SA*, the air principle, is the impersonal infinity. When sound takes place in the external plane, it becomes *SA*, which represents manifestation. The first part of the mantra expands toward heaven. By repeating the sound *SA*, it becomes a turning point, causing the spirit to descend from above into matter in order to animate and vitalize it with healing and life. In other words, the second part of the mantra brings the healing qualities of the superior world back down to the Earth. The last stanza of the emerald tablet from the great Hermes Trismegistus, which reveals the secret of healing and order in the material plane, is followed in this mantra. It reads, *"Ascend with great sagacity from Earth to Heaven, and then again descend to Earth, and unite together the powers of things superior and inferior. Thus you will obtain the glory of the whole world and obscurity will fly away from you."*

The secret is adaptation, transforming one thing into another thing. *Ra Ma Da Sa* transforms an imbalanced, unhealthy body into a harmonious, healthy one. As with the Star of David, a symbol of two interlaced triangles, this mantra interlinks spirit with matter.

SAY comes after *SA*, and represents the totality of experience. *SO* is the personal sense of identity. *HUNG* is the infinite, vibrating and real. The sound *Tho*, or *SO*, sounded in the note of F sharp in the middle octave of the piano keyboard, stimulates the thyroid gland so vital to good healthy living. The thyroid gland controls and sustains physical development, and affects the learning and responsive energies of both mind and muscle. In addition, a normal thyroid regulates the secretion of chemicals, such as iodine and arsenic, in the system. Spiritually speaking, the thyroid controls the rapidity of the interchange of objective and subconscious impressions, even though it is not the place where the exchange actually takes place. *Tho* helps to bring out our sympathetic feeling toward our fellow man, and it assists in creating the power of adaptability.

HUNG is suggestive of *Hu*, which is the life of God in every thing and every being. The *NG* causes the sound in *HUNG* to stimulate the divine glands. The sound of the breath is *SO HUNG*. *SO* is the inhale, *HUNG* the exhale. The two qualities of *SO HUNG* together mean, "I am Thou." As stated earlier, when you chant this mantra, you expand toward the infinite and merge back with the finite. *AUM OM*, or *HUNG*, is a potent sound associated with the creative forces. It affects the pineal gland responsible for transforming intelligence from the spiritual to the objective consciousness so that you are able to access many of the impressions gained in previous incarnations. Most people have forgotten that their essence is with the infinite, unlimited creative power of the cosmos.

When a person goes within himself and consciously experiences his own beauty, he touches his divinity. He is then able to reunite his destiny with his highest potential.

Throughout the ages, yoga and Kabbalah masters have known that words and thoughts can program our bodies. Indeed, from an esoteric or spiritual point of view it is entirely normal and natural that our DNA reacts to language, especially when it comes in the form of a mantra, or sound current, such as *Ra Ma Da Sa*. "In the beginning was the Word." If everything comes from the Word, it follows that the Word can correct anything. This ancient knowledge is now being confirmed and explained by scientists. Interestingly, only 10% of our DNA is used to build proteins. The remaining 90% is erroneously considered junk. It is this subset of DNA, of particular interest to western researchers, which is now being examined and categorized.

Our DNA is not only responsible for the construction of our bodies. It also stores data and communication. Russian linguists have found that the genetic code—especially in the apparently "useless" 90%—follows the same rules as human language. It follows then, as a wealth of scientific evidence now suggests, that DNA can be influenced and reprogrammed via words, sound, and frequencies without removing and/or replacing single genes. This discovery has far reaching implications for physical healing and the world of western medicine. Living chromosomes function just like a holographic computer using endogenous DNA laser radiation. In living tissue, DNA substance will always react to language-modulated laser rays if the proper frequencies (sounds) are being used. This scientifically explains why affirmations, hypnosis, mantra, and the like can have such strong effects on humans and their bodies. Herein lies an amazing, potentially world-transforming revolution in medicinal healing. By substituting vibration (sound frequencies) and language for the archaic procedure of cutting, you can affect the DNA. Again, this highlights the fact that it is possible for one to transfer a perfect pattern of health, via a healing vibration, into every cell of an unhealthy body. In other words, those who are properly trained can restore and maintain health by transmitting a healing vibration pattern to the DNA information pattern.

It cannot be stressed enough that listening to or chanting *Ra Ma Da Sa* is not only a good means of practical, preventative self-healthcare, but it will also aid in the assurance of a healthier life. It can help preserve the body and pave the way toward a positive mental projection. Chanting or listening to this mantra set to this classical tune will drive out depression and revibrate your life. It is timeless. It has worked in the past, it works now, and it will work in the future. There is no time, no place, no space, and no condition attached to this mantra. Use it everyday to burn away the seed of disease. Offer it to others. If you work with it, it will work for you. In moments of anxiety, despair, fear or worry, let it be your safeguard. It will give you a strong sense of your own centeredness. This mantra is a pure divine thought. When you think pure thoughts and are mentally strong, you cannot suffer the painful effects of bad karma or disease. A regular practice of listening to this CD or chanting along with it is like praying unceasingly. When you continuously pray and meditate, you go into the land of Light, where all troubles disappear.

The Lion's Heart Series Reference Guide

A (1st time) Open hands*

B (2nd time) Touch tips of thumb, ring and pinkie fingers

C (3rd time)
Thumb to index fingertip

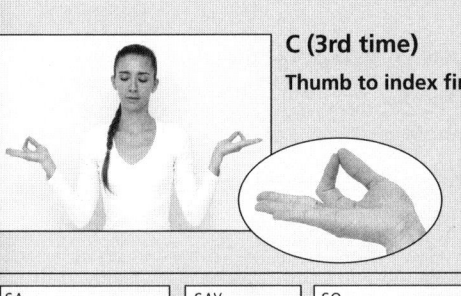

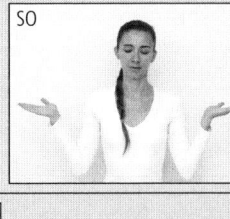

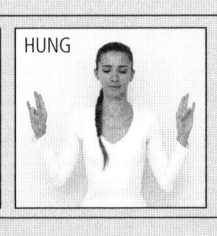

SA	SAY	SO	HUNG	
				* Ravi mudra (thumb to ring finger) only for A

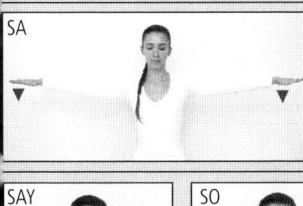

SA — Start both hands face up, then down; repeat sequence through the phrase (total of 4x each direction)

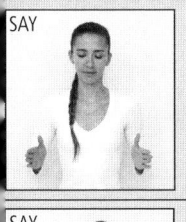

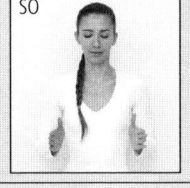

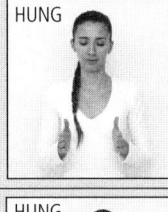

SAY / SO / HUNG — Open 4 segments / Close 4 segments

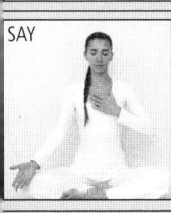

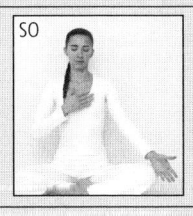

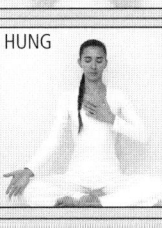

SAY / SO / HUNG — Start right hand to heart; left hand open on knee

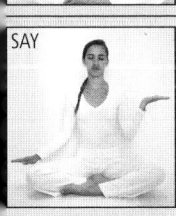

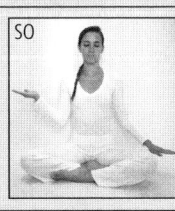

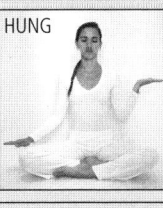

SAY / SO / HUNG — Start right hand up; left down

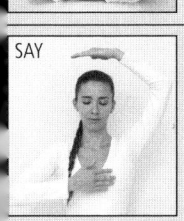

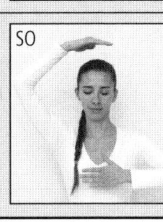

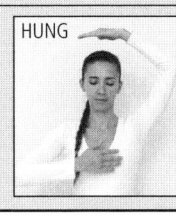

SAY / SO / HUNG — Start right hand over head; left in front of heart

The Lion's Heart Mudra Series with Ra Ma Da Sa Sa Say So Hung

The Lion's Heart Series builds a tremendously powerful and protective aura. During this meditation the entire body is revitalized and renewed. It may be done with the mantra *Ra Ma Da Sa Sa Say So Hung* (we recommend the Rootlight CDs *Ra Ma Da Sa* or track 4 of *The Healing Spirit of Ra Ma Da Sa*). This series is effective when performed one time through (A, B and C) on a daily basis. For a more permanent effect, 11 minutes daily is sufficient. For serious cases, do the series for 31 minutes a day.

POSITION:
Sit in a comfortable meditative pose, such as Easy Pose, with the spine and neck straight. The shoulders are relaxed. The eyes are closed, focused at the brow point.

MUDRAS:
A: First time through the series
Palms open and fingers extended.
The only exception in the "A" series is position **A8** where the thumb and ring fingertips touch (Ravi Mudra) and the other fingers stretch straight up.

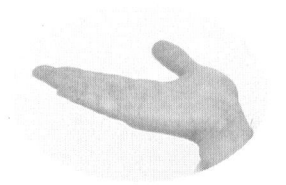

B: Second time through the series
Silver Triangle (Thumb to the tips of the ring and pinkie fingers; the index and middle fingers are straight side by side)

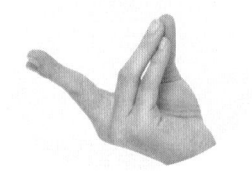

C: Third time through the series
Gyan Mudra (Thumb to index finger; the other fingers extended)

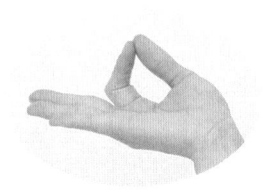

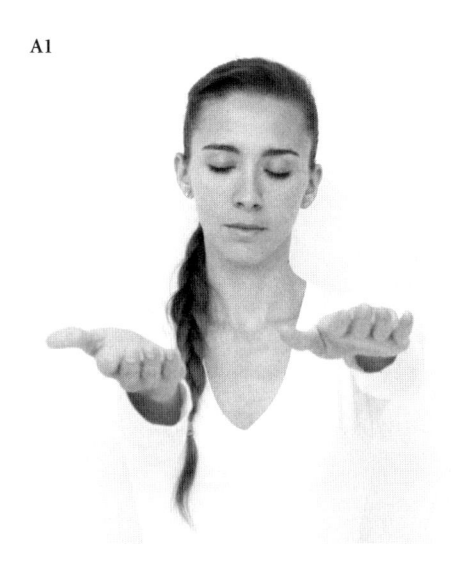

Position 1: "RA"

The arms are extended directly in front of you parallel to each other and parallel to the ground. The right palm faces up, and the left palm faces down.

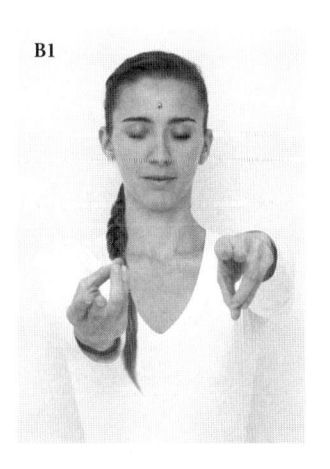

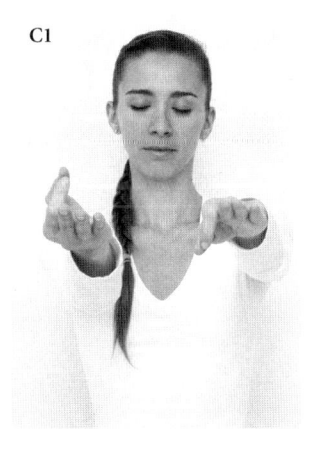

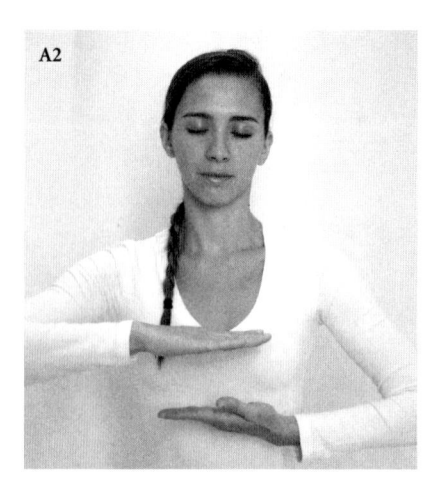

POSITION 2: "MA"

Bend the elbows so the hands are about one inch from the torso. The right palm faces down, and the left faces up, with the hands parallel to each other, approximately 8 inches apart.

The empty space encompasses the distance from the heart to the solar plexus area, as if you are holding a ball of light.

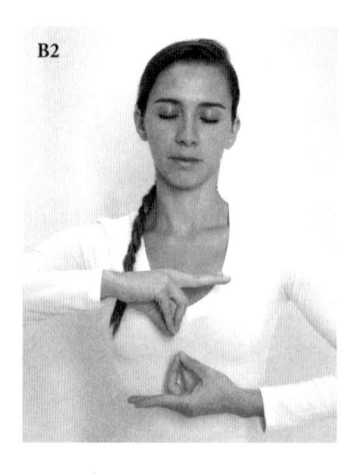

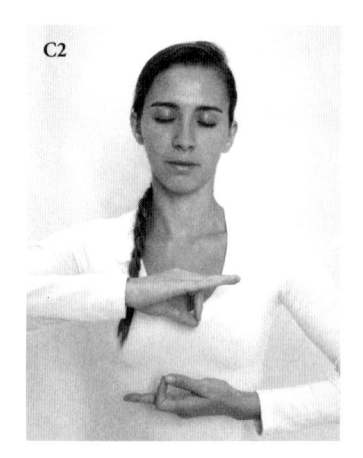

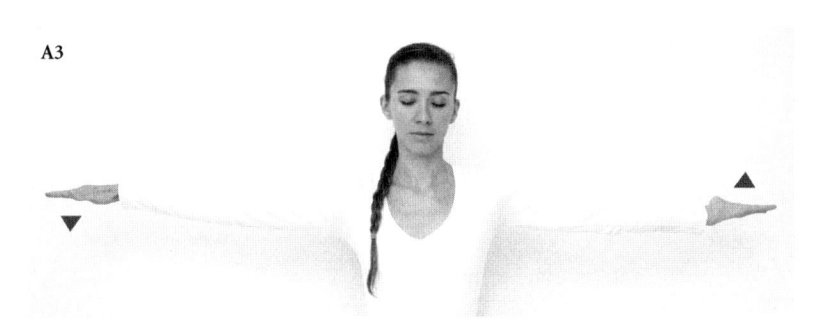

Position 3: "DA"

Unfold the arms directly to the side until they are completely extended, parallel to the ground. The right palm stays facing down and left palm facing up.

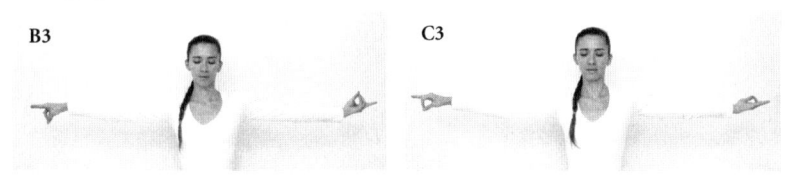

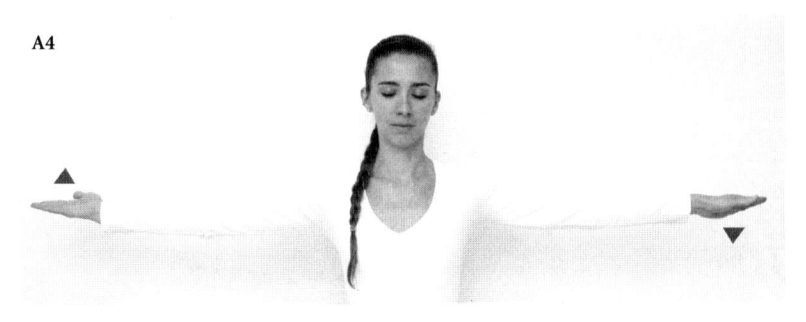

Position 4: "SA"

Arms stay in this position, but the palms switch; right palm faces up and left palm faces down.

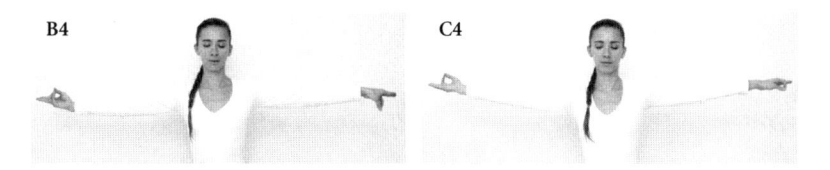

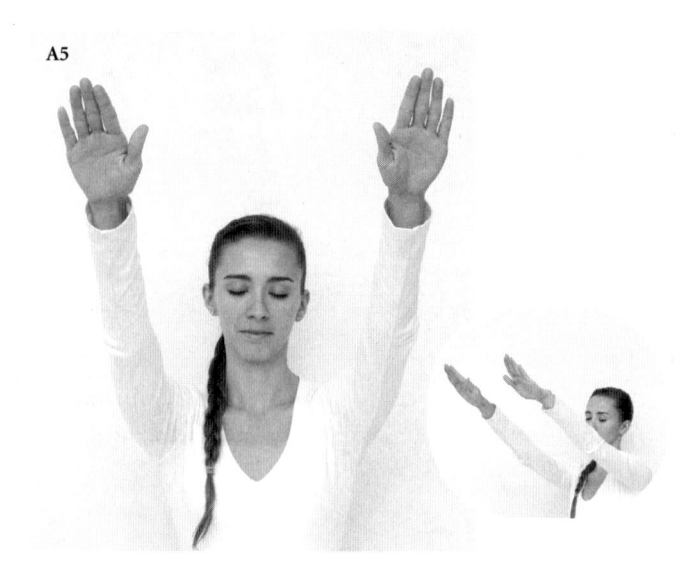

POSITION 5: "SA"
Extend the arms, parallel to each other, 60° in front of the body, palms facing down.

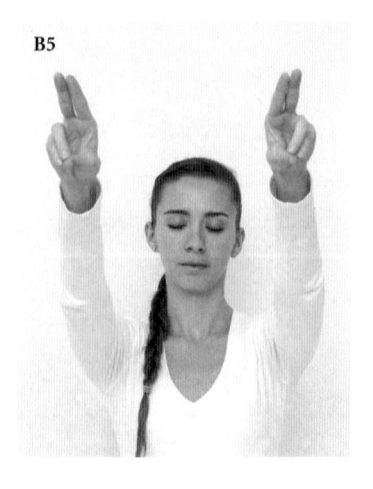

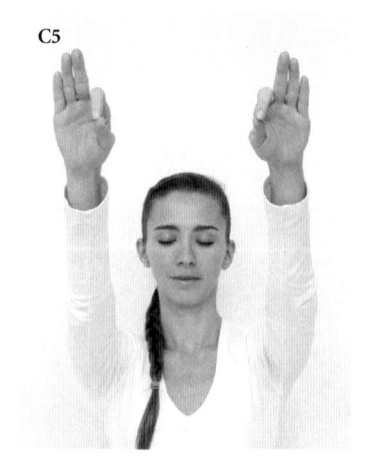

A6

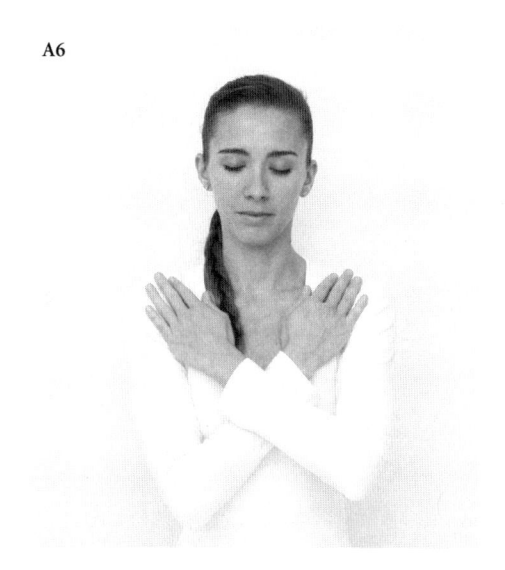

POSITION 6: "SAY"
Cross the hands over the heart; left hand over right.

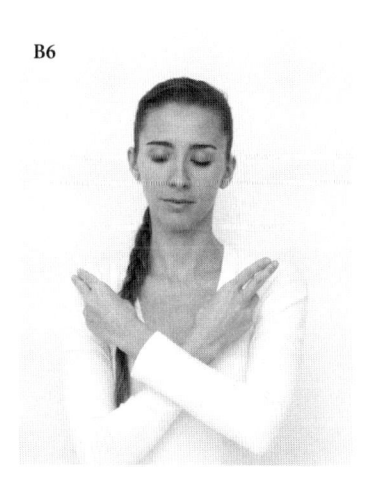

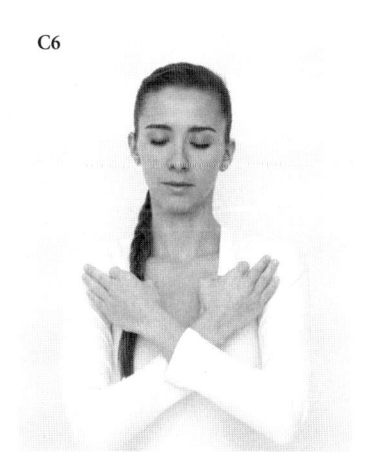

B6

C6

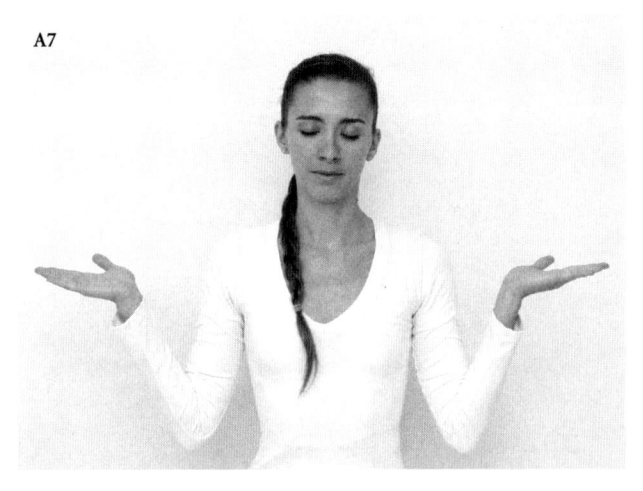

POSITION 7: "SO"
The arms are bent at the sides, elbows relaxed; the palms are angled towards the body at approximately 60°, so that they are slightly facing up.

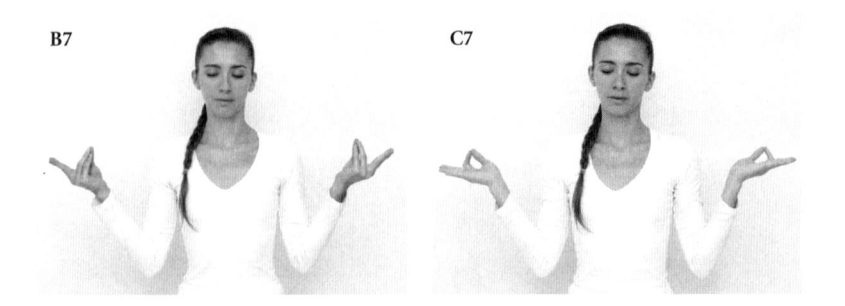

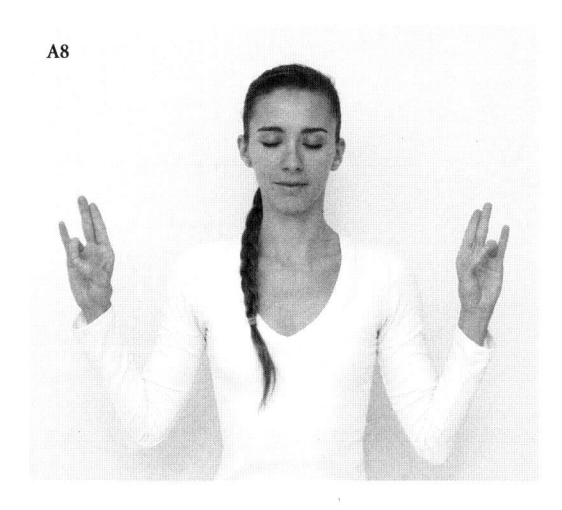

POSITION 8: "HUNG"

The arms stay down by the sides, but palms face forward and the hands are in Ravi Mudra (tip of the thumb is touching the tip of the ring finger). *Note: Ravi Mudra is used only in series A. For series B and C, you will maintain the specific mudra for that series.*

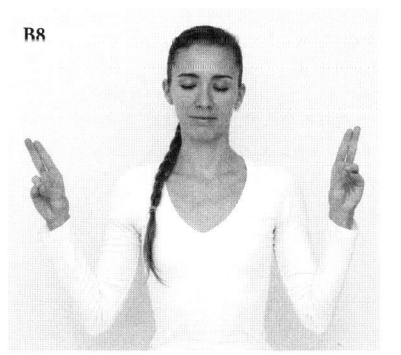

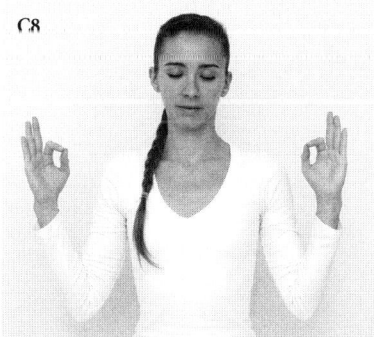

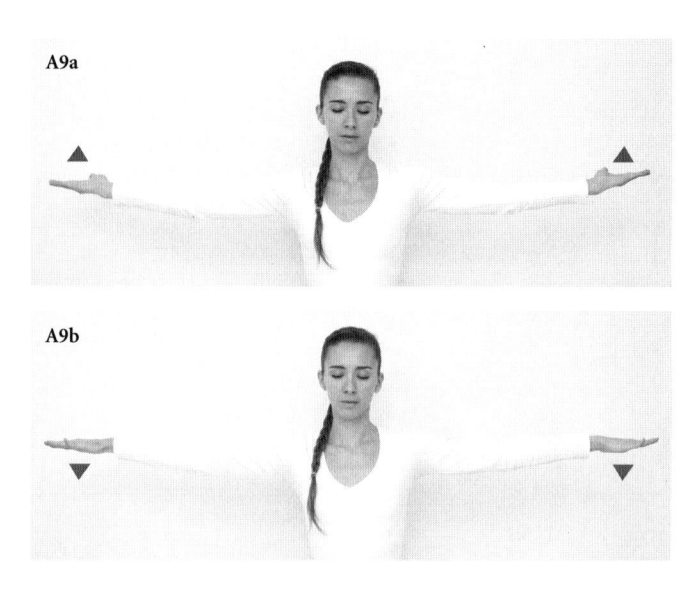

POSITION 9:

A. "RA" — Extend arms straight out to the side as in #3; this time both palms face up.
B. "MA" — Palms face down.
C. "DA" — Palms face up.
D. "SA" — Palms face down.
E. "SA" — Palms face up.
F. "SAY" — Palms face down.
G. "SO" — Palms face up.
H. "HUNG" — Palms face down.

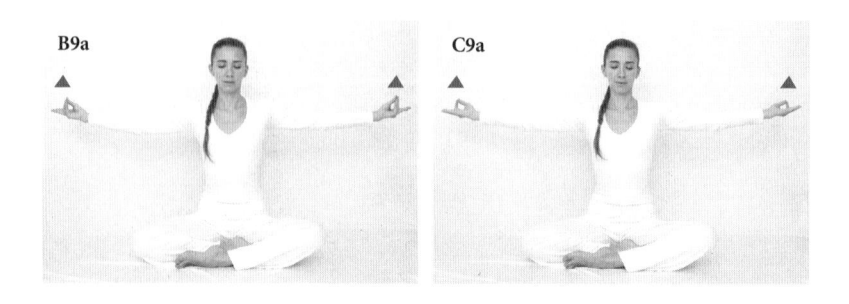

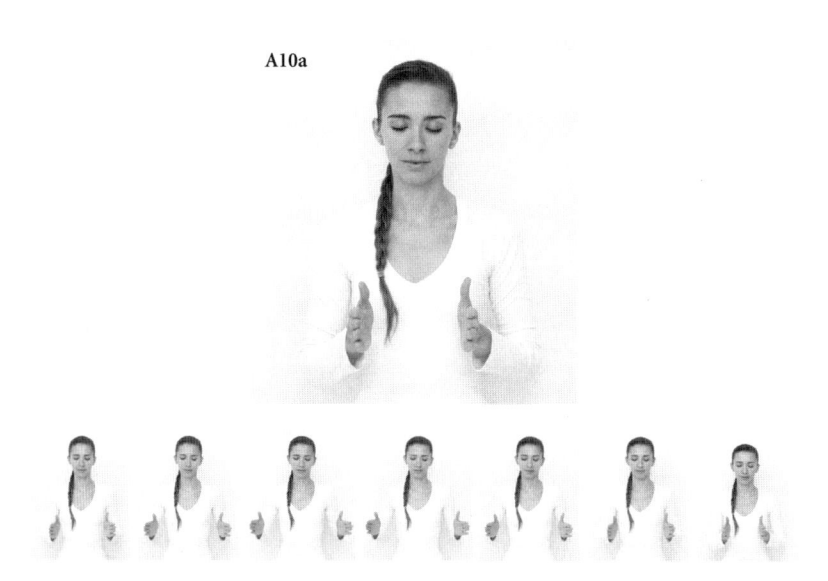

POSITION 10:
GENTLY MOVE HANDS APART IN 4 SEGMENTS AND BACK IN 4 SEGMENTS

A. "RA" — Hands are in Middle Pillar mudra (palms facing each other in front of the solar plexus approximately 6 inches apart).

B. "MA" — Hands stay in Middle Pillar, but move slightly apart approximately 1-2 inches.

C. "DA" — Hands move apart more, approximately 1-2 inches.

D. "SA" — Hands move even more, to end approx. 10-12 inches apart.

E. "SA" — Hands move in slightly closer, approx. 1-2 inches.

F. "SAY" — Hands move closer, approximately 1-2 inches.

G. "SO" — Hands move closer, approximately 1-2 inches.

H. "HUNG" — Hands are back to original position, about 6 inches apart.

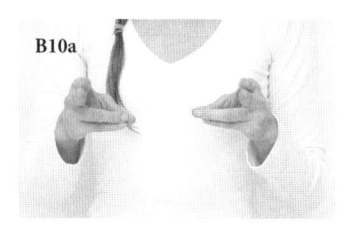

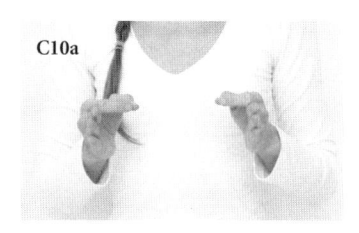

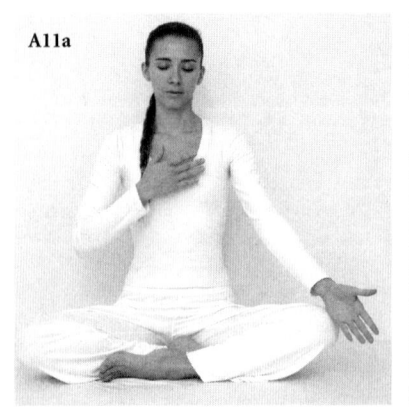

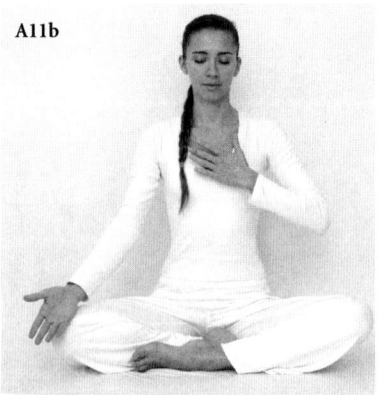

Position 11:
Slowly fan the heart with alternating hands

A. **"RA"** — Start with the right palm fanning the heart, coming within an inch of the chest, left arm extended to the knee.

B. **"MA"** — Left palm moves to the heart, right arm extends to the knee.

Complete the phrase while alternating between right and left.

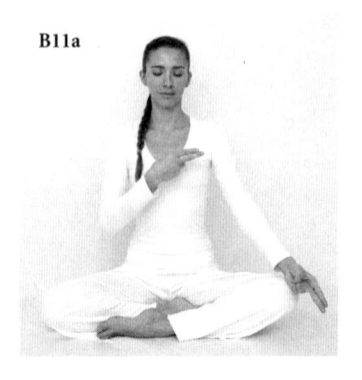

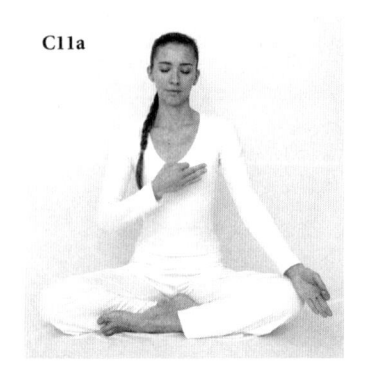

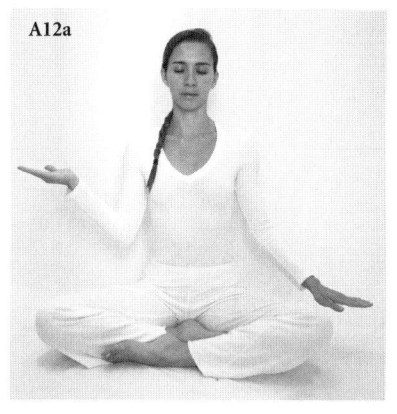

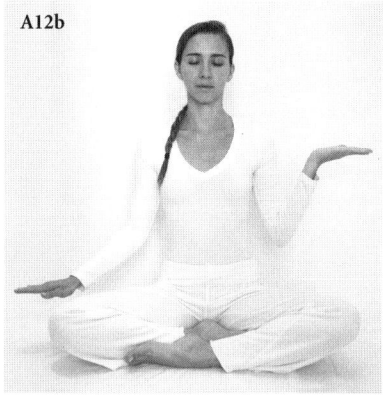

Position 12:
Slowly alternate hands at your side

A. "RA" — Start with the right palm facing up, the upper right arm is bent and the elbow relaxed near the side of the body; left arm is slightly bent, elbow pointing back, palm is facing down.

B. "MA" — Arms alternate so that left hand rises, palm facing up, and the right palm faces down and arm extends down, creating a mirror image of (A).

Complete the phrase while alternating between right and left.

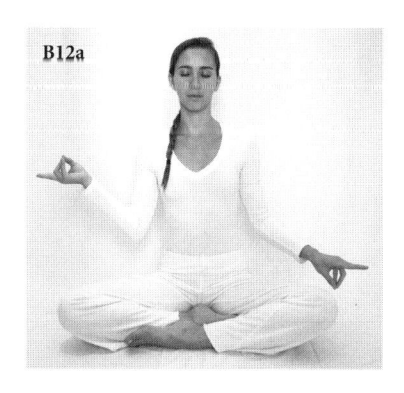

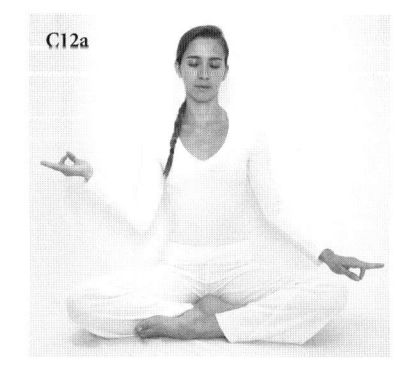

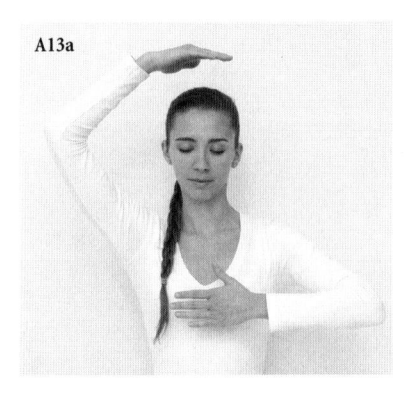

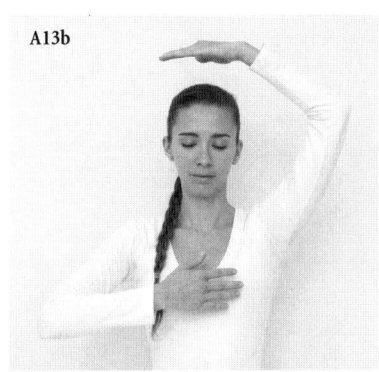

Position 13:
Slowly alternate hands while sweeping energy between the crown and the heart

A. "RA" — Start with the right hand slightly above the crown chakra, palm facing down, elbow out to the side; the left arm is bent, elbow out to the side, palm facing the heart close to the chest.

B. "MA" — Switch arms, so the left palm gracefully rises to hover just above the crown chakra, sweeping slightly behind the head, positioned where the right palm was. The right palm directs energy from crown along the center (moon) line until it rests slightly in front of the heart, positioned where the left palm was.

Complete the phrase while alternating between right and left.

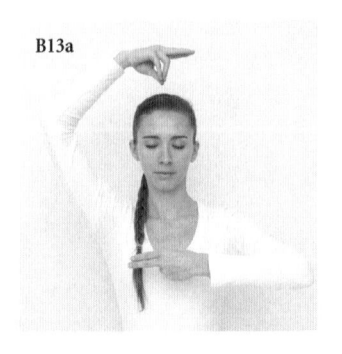

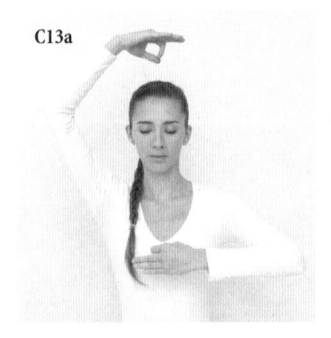

21

THE BONES

THERE IS AN ADMIRABLE SUBSTANCE that contains all power, all virtue, and is the essence and foundation of the light being. It is an indestructible substance endowed with great power for those who know how to develop and use it. This germ of immortality hidden inside the human bones is imperishable and indestructible, and it cannot be dissolved. When man passes away, this substance does not die, nor does it fly away or go into syncope, even if the person has been cremated. This substance can neither be burned nor consumed. It cannot be broken, and it endures forever based upon the purity of the behavior, thoughts and speech of the person while he was alive. It is a celestial substance, the subject of all wonder, the very foundation of man's being. It is on the earth and in the heavens, yet unknown by most people. This substance can be found in the human bones. The human bones and particularly the twenty-six vertebrae form the perfect expression of the one Law of Manifestation behind of all life. This life must therefore follow universal stages of unfoldment.

The bones and twenty-six vertebrae must be recognized as the symbol and example of the Great Divine Mystery of the manifested Godhead, and universal law of manifestation so exact and mathematically correct in every detail that it must be an expression of a fundamental infinite truth, the manifestation of God in His Works. The twenty-six vertebrae, as the Sun of the skeletal system, are the actual manifested result of a higher and more divine truth, the One eternal and absolute creative

God in the midst of His creation. The human bones and especially the twenty-six vertebrae are not only the nucleus of the body, but they are also a material expression of this One eternal Godhead, while the rest of the physical vehicle is but the limiting body in which the spine must do the will of He who sent them forth. The human skeleton behaves like the seed of the fruit that is the human being. Nothing is more important than the seed in the fruit. For nature, the essential is in the seed. Nature is only interested in the seed which behaves like the spirit, and the flesh is the space where life circulates. The human skin is the material envelope of the physical body. The proof that cosmic intelligence is not very attached to the physical body is that the latter is left to die and be buried, whereas the immortal spirit returns to the celestial regions, and the bones endure.

The human skeleton supports the human body. Without it, we would be reduced to a fleshy blob. Working with the muscular system, the skeletal system allows us to move while acting as the storehouse of calcium and other important minerals, and manufacturing blood cells. The human skeleton also works to protect our delicate, vital internal organs, preventing them from being damaged. There are two major systems of bones in the human body, the axial skeleton and the appendicular skeleton. The axial skeleton is comprised of the 80 bones in the skull, ribs, and sternum. The appendicular skeleton has 126 bones from the shoulders, pelvis, and attached limbs. Our joints connect bones to other bones, and there are many different types including: fixed joints, such as those found in the skull; hinged joints, such as those found in the fingers and toes; and ball-and-socket joints, such as those found in the shoulders and hips. In addition, each bone is comprised of three major sections, the compact bone, the soft bone marrow that produces red blood cells, and the sponge bone. The longest bone in our bodies is the femur, or thighbone. The smallest bone is the stirrup bone inside the ear.

While men and women have slightly different skeletons, men have slightly thicker, longer legs and arms, women have a wider, more spacious pelvis through which babies travel when they are born. All human beings, regardless of gender, class, creed, or color have white bones. This is due to the fact that all human beings can be traced back to one single cell, one single DNA, and One God. White is the color of the Sun. In it you find the seven colors of the spectrum, or the seven Archangels. Therefore, our bones, the unseen structure and foundation of the body, are the seven colors of the rainbow merged in one unified color, white. We are born with approximately 300 bones, but as we grow up some bones fuse together, leaving us with 206. The number 206 reduces to 8, the number of Saturn, the Lord of Karma and planet of structure and spirituality. Eight is the number of healing and spirituality. It is no accident that the number of bones found in the human body is the same as the number of Saturn, structure, healing, and spirituality, for our bones provide our bodies with structure and contain an unknown spiritual, healing essence. Again, they are the foundation of the body. On the Tree of Life, Yesod, the Moon, stands for foundation. Yesod is the foundation or Basis, represented by *El Chai*, the Mighty Living One, and *Shaddai*, and among the angels by *Aishim*, the Flames. It is the realm of the astral light and is responsible for the vital, life-ether necessary for vivification of the material body and reproduction. Yesod is also responsible for the chemical ether necessary for maintenance of the physical world, represented by Malkuth. Working with Yesod allows you to control the material world, just as working with the bones allows you to take care of the physical body and material life. Both Yesod and the bones, then, are our foundation and the point of balance and stability on the Tree of Life and in the human edifice. Remove Yesod and the whole Tree falls apart. Remove the bones and the whole body falls apart. Yesod is the subtle fundament upon which the physical world is based. It corresponds to the astral plane. The astral light is an omnipresent and all-permeating fluid or medium of extremely subtle matter; substance in a highly tenuous state, electric and magnetic in constitution, which is the model upon which the physical world is built. It is the endless and changeless, ebb and flow of the world's forces that, in the last resort, guarantee the stability of the world and provide its foundation.

Yesod is the stable foundation, this changeless ebb and flow of astral forces, and the universal reproductive power in nature. Everything shall return to its foundation from which it has proceeded. All marrow seed and energy are gathered in its place. Therefore, all potentialities which exist go out through this place. Its Hindu equivalent is Ganesha who breaks down all obstacles and supports the universe. Its Roman equivalent is Diana who is the princess of light and represents the Moon. The astral light, which is sphere of Yesod, is also referred to as the *Anima Mundi* or the Soul of the world. It is the collective unconscious.

The number eight, which is the number of Saturn, leads us on the Tree of Life to the sphere Binah. Binah is Shakti, the universal electric vital power which unites and brings together all forms, the constructive power of the Divine that carries out in the formation of all things. Binah reveals to us the mysteries of destiny, because it enlightens us about the Law of Cause and Effect. The third Sephirah of the Kabbalah Tree of Life is a feminine passive potency, called Binah, the Understanding, who is co-equal with Chokmah. Thus this Sephirah completes and makes evident the supernal Trinity. It is also called Ama, Mother, and Aima, the great productive Mother, who is eternally conjoined with the Father, for the maintenance of the universe in order. Therefore she is the most evident form in whom we can know the Father, and therefore she is worthy of all honor. She is the supernal Mother, co-equal with Chokmah, and the great feminine form of God, the Elohim, in whose image man and woman are created, and according to the teachings of the Kabbalah, equal before God. Aima is the woman described in the Apocalypse. This third Sephirah is also sometimes called the Great Sea. To her are attributed the Divine names, Aralim, the Thrones. She is the supernal Mother, as distinguished from Malkuth, the inferior Mother, Bride and Queen. You will find the elements that will allow you to understand why fate and destiny behave the way they do in Binah. Again, in Binah you have the angelic hierarchy made up of the *Aralims* also called Thrones. These are what St. John saw in his vision in the form of the twenty-four Elders. These Elders are known as the Lord of Destiny, because they are the one who examine the way each person has lived in previous lives and determine his destiny according to his merits. Their decrees are carried out by the angels of Chesed—the Hasmalim who dispense rewards—or the angels of Geburah—the Seraphim who administer punishment. Chesed is Mercy or Love, also called Gedulah, Greatness or Magnificence;

a masculine potency represented by the Divine Name Al, El, the Mighty One, and the angelic name, Chashmalim, Scintillating Flames. Geburah is strength or fortitude; or Din, Deen, Justice; represented by the divine names Elohim Gibor, Eloh, and the angelic name Seraphim. This Sephirah is also called Pachad, or Fear.

Destiny is an archetypal form, and each person lives his life according to the form destiny assigned to him. The twenty-four Elders from Binah represent the divine tribunal that decrees the forms of human destinies, and the physical forms we see on earth are simply a reflection of those who have been decreed on high. One of these forms is projected in the womb of every pregnant woman, and it is this form which provides the basis of the work of gestation. Once these forms are decreed, there is no changing them. They descend on the material plane on which they take physical form. Destiny can only be changed by changing the archetypes. There is no other way. Everything is ordained in such a way that what must be will be. In order to change one's destiny, one must reach the region beyond Binah. In other words, the regions that are above and beyond destiny, the region of Chokmah and Kether. Our fate is the consequence of our past incarnations. All our difficulties are problems that we have been given to resolve; they offer the most effective means of evolution.

The inflexible character of Binah, which is represented by the garland of skulls that hangs from the neck of the Hindu Kali to display her terrible destructive side, is seen also in the symbolism of Saturn, which is portrayed as an old man or sometimes as a skeleton carrying a scythe. The scythe of Saturn represents time which destroys everything, and the skeleton represents eternity, that which resists the attack of time. Saturn represents both aspects. Beyond the domain of the flesh, the world of external appearances that is continually being destroyed by time (the scythe) is the indestructible skeleton (eternity). It takes a strong spiritual practice, many sincere prayers and meditation to understand how to make the passage from time to eternity.

It is also important to add here that according to the Kabbalah each soul has two angels, a good and an evil one. From Ruach (reason) and Nephesh (passion) influenced by the good aspiration of Neshamah, proceeds Michael, the good angel of the soul. From Nephesh dominating Ruach and uninfluenced by the good aspiration of Neshamah, proceeds Shamael, the evil angel of the soul.

Thus the duality of man is explained. Reason controlling the passions creates a good angel Michael, literally a force which each soul draws from the sun and entitizes, and which becomes a reliable helper towards higher development.

When passion dominates or is excused and its indulgence is argued away by reason, it creates an entitized evil angel or genius, Shamael, which is always ready to give a plausible excuse or reason why black should be called white and evil, good. Man's personality has an image which is double, since it can reflect either Michael or Shamael.

Those who are spiritually evolved and have disformed bodies or repulsive features, have in some incarnation permitted Shamael to rule and find expression in their lives. Therefore, they must bear his imprint until the rule of Michael can transmute it in his beautiful image. The choice is whether we let Michael or Shamael rule our lives and make his imprint in our bodies. True beauty is an expression of soul development. Those who today have beautiful bodies and evil minds are those who in the past have allowed Michael to rule, but who today are allowing the imprint of Shamael to take over that of Michael.

A change in one's fate can be made through the Word of God. A man of God speaks the Word of God, and the Word of God is what opens the heart of the ignorant person to Godhood.

22

HARMONYUM: THE UNKNOWN MEDICINE

The invisible nature of man is as vast as his ability to comprehend it and is as measureless as his thoughts. The man of today is a ternary composition, made up of the spirit which emanates from the breast of Divinity, of which it is the image, and which is indestructible like him; of the soul or perishable passive animal life, emanated by secondary agents; of a material body formed of the three corporeal principles. The animal is only a binary composition, formed of the passive soul and a material body, neither of which bear the indelible nature of life and indestructibility, and only have momentary action. The indestructible form of creative man was created by the will of the Creator without any physical working of matter, such as was necessary for the material corporeal forms to which the children of man have been subjected, since his fall. Man is not the insignificant creature that he appears to be; his physical body is not the true measure of his real self. The fingers of his mind reach out and grasp the stars; his spirit mingles with the throbbing life of Cosmos itself. He who increases his spiritual understanding gradually incorporates within himself the unseen elements of the universe, for the unknown is merely that which is yet to be included within the consciousness of a human.

Harmonyum healing regenerates the entire human psyche through the vivifying impact of Christic love, so as to cause one to unfold those latent powers and faculties whereby one may master the secrets of the seven spheres. These spheres symbolize the seven Elohim expressed through the seven sacred powers of the cosmos, the seven nature notes and the seven colors into which the one white light (or the Yod) is broken up. Full regeneration cannot be attained without the life-giving and life-restoring touch of true love, for Divine Love is the creative force that drives the vital breath in both the individual and the Divine. Regeneration through Christic love involves the sublimation of vice into virtue. For the majority of human beings, vice is more attractive than the austere beauty of virtue. Remember, however, that while vice may appear more satisfactory in the short run, virtue ensures victory in the long run. A chain of flowers is more difficult to break than one of iron. Virtue is not simply a lofty, unapproachable concept; it requires our focused attention and our judicious action in the heat of the moment. When we effectively direct our actions in a moment where opposing passions co-exist, we create a powerful balance. That is the great secret of virtuous living: we balance the scales of our emotions and desires with the elements that govern the situation and achieve a neutral outcome that addresses the higher good.

Movement is life; balance carries movement forward. When we are virtuous, we are living in the flow of balance, a flow of movement. Conversely, immobility is death. When we are stuck in our perspective and unable to recognize anything outside of ourselves, we experience a kind of ongoing death. When we ignore our deepest instincts, the conflict we feel from the lack of natural balance within us often produces health issues that lead to our destruction. When we use our free will intelligently and virtuously, we liberate ourselves from the fatality of circumstances that could have been easily avoided. When we reconcile reason and feeling, energy and gentleness of spirit, we live in moral balance that is the scientific basis of living. The instinctive existence of animals reminds us to live effortlessly in the moment. In certain species, animal instinct is sharper and better attuned than human instinct. Nature has provided for the preservation of animals and man by endowing each with instincts; however, man has the responsibility of utilizing his God-given intelligence to discern as well as intuit the roadmap of life. Man is an intelligent spiritual being who must learn to honor his role in Nature's design by respecting the moral balance within himself and serving as an example of the Christic force in action. True regeneration is the act of being reborn in the Spirit whereby the body and soul are penetrated by the heat of Divine Love and the light of Divine intelligence that emanates from the Divine fire held within self-consciousness and self-knowledge.

Harmonyum works on the body of resurrection by raising the vibratory frequency of the entire material body and infusing it with sufficient energy so that it may become the breath of life. What makes the resurrection body different is that while it can and does exist within the material world, it is free from material limitation. This perfect body was, or is, essentially a quintessence differentiated into subtle and simple elements. Conversely, the physical body is contaminated by the grosser elements. Harmonyum is the bridge between the body of the flesh and the body of the resurrection, igniting the fire within for divine healing to begin to regenerate and accelerate the processes of the entire developmental spiritual system.

Harmonyum not only works on the spiritual and physical bodies, but above all, it affects that part of the human body that corresponds to Daath, the mysterious, unknown eleventh Sephirah of the Kabbalah Tree of Life. It is here that the tidal forces of positive and negative intertwine to be used for the benefit of the physical developmental system. Daath is the storehouse of all the energy of the physical universe and its developmental system counterpart. Daath is the cosmic abyss which contains all the records of the past—all the archives of the cosmos from the beginning of time. It is the primal chaos, over which hovers the spirit of God. Daath also holds the key to the Fall of Man, for it was through this Sephirah that Temptation came to Adam and Eve. The serpent was, in fact, Shamael, that extremely powerful spirit who persuaded Adam and Eve to eat the fruit of the Tree of Knowledge of Good and Evil. As punishment for their decision to ignore God's law, they were expelled from Paradise.

Before the Fall, Daath was the point at which the symbolic River Naher, the descending current of energy from the Supernals, was divided into the four rivers of Eden (ether divides into the four elements). After the Fall, Daath became the highest reach of the Dragon, the point at which the waters of Life were corrupted by the dragon's venom into waters of Death. At Daath, too, the four Cherubim and the Flaming Sword keep watch at the gate of the Higher Eden; they guard against the unbalanced powers below and serve as a revelation of the way in which those powers can be overcome. From this perspective, Daath's role as a barrier has been heightened by the Fall, while its role as a point of contact has been lessened—at least from a human perspective. Still, the Gate of the Abyss can be opened, and that opening is the supreme practical work of the Universal Kabbalist.

Daath allows one to receive the knowledge which comes from experience and conscious realization of the experience. Through the experience in real life of the Wisdom which comes from Chokmah, one achieves the understanding that comes from Binah and gains the healing knowledge that is the spiritual succor of existence. You cannot integrate the divine spiritual wisdom unless you create within yourself the capacity to understand it. Once comprehended, it becomes knowledge that lives and breathes within you and which can be shared with authenticity.

Harmonyum bestows upon you the untroubled peace that moves you to face your darkness and transmute it into light. Daath is a link between the conscious self and the transcendent spirit, the medium through which all contact with the Higher Genius must take place. The opening of Daath permits the return of our awareness to its transcendent source, and the full opening of Daath involves the highest levels of spiritual attainment. A partial opening of the gate, on the other hand, can take place on a much more modest level of development.

Receiving Harmonyum progressively opens the gates to Daath, the unknown. The gradual opening of the Daath center is of the highest importance to the Universal Kabbalist for two reasons. First, the interface between Ruach and Neshamah is also said to be the interface between the parts of the self that perish along with the death of the physical body and those parts that do not. As that interface becomes more active, more of the structure of the conscious self is preserved through the stages of death and rebirth, and lessons learned in one life can be carried over to others with less difficulty. Second, the interface between Ruach and Neshamah is a source of power, as well as of spiritual knowledge. Ruach is the root of outward consciousness and allows one to become aware through forms and their expression. It is all conscious and unconscious mental activity. Ruach is the energy that gives rise to thoughts that will be brought into action. It rules the personality. Ruach is the second part of the soul to enter the body, which it does with the first breath at birth. Neshamah is the source of knowledge and intelligence. It is the highest state of consciousness. Also, each of us has a guardian angel, which is the pure Spirit commissioned by the Eternal to look after us for the Reconciliation of our spiritual body. Harmonyum creates a platform for you to connect with your guardian angel. It causes the God of mercy to allow your guardian to come to the aid of your soul, whenever it is in danger of yielding to darkness.

It is vital to keep in mind that we initiate the force of reconstruction within by working with the universe. The universe is kept intact by the energy of Love, and Love is the one quality necessary for the advancement of human beings in virtue and truth. Indeed, Divine Love is at the root of all healing and growth. While intelligence and activity are necessary in order to grow and accomplish the work of man, Love is the force that precedes, and thus supports, intelligence and activity. When this Love energy flows through our bodies properly, we experience happiness and health. Conversely, when such energy is cut off and replaced with the energy of hurt feelings, emotional entanglements, resentment, fear, and frustration, we experience varying degrees of disharmony and disease. Harmonyum is one of the few healing systems known to impart the nurturing, unconditional Love that surrounds and supports the universe. During a session, the recipient automatically experiences the restoration of the natural flow of Love in the body that nurtures the organs, as well as an increase in pranic supply to the cells. Harmonyum is able to achieve such healing results because as its techniques melt physical tension, the recipient's spiritual body is able to release healing prana. He/she moves into a healing space as Love washes away all resentments, fears, and doubts.

Unknown to most, there are two types of fire, that which is inferior and that which is superior. Inferior fire consumes by making a bad fecundation, while superior fire creates, produces, and gives birth. Harmonyum works with the superior fire in order to heal. Receiving a

Harmonyum treatment manifests the Light in the consciousness of the recipient, dynamically expanding his/her awareness of that Light. This new awareness is the realization of oneself in alignment with the flow of life. One begins to understand the fundamental fact that we are all God, because God is within each of us. In turn, we begin to recreate our existence in accordance with our True Will rather than our ego consciousness. Consistent Harmonyum treatments help recipients reach a high state of consciousness. It is even possible, via Harmonyum, to neutralize the seven negative karmic influences and control the automatic life process, for Harmonyum causes individuals to become more aware. With increased awareness, one can positively alter mental attitudes and speech patterns. In other words, Harmonyum expands one's awareness so that you are able to recognize how the law of cause and effect impacts your life. By changing attitudes and behaviors, you can control and even undo the damage caused by living in disharmony. In addition, you are able to cultivate the power to choose how you will think and act, rather than relying on automatic reactions. This, in turn, allows you to replace the habits that keep you trapped in the cycle of negative patterns. You begin to understand the intimate connection between your body and mind. Your body responds, both positively and negatively, to your given set of attitudes. Maintain positive attitudes, and your health will be bolstered.

In other words, Harmonyum will turn your body into a lighthouse. This transcendental healing system, which is born out of Universal Kabbalah and also known as Bio-Metaphysical Medicine, is the healing system for this age and beyond. Harmonyum heals all the cavities that can accumulate in the auric field. This gentle transformative process eliminates negativity and discordant energy throughout your system, canceling out self-abusive patterns that also externally attract bad luck and challenges to your health. One treatment can be as effective as years worth of therapy in that it encourages the subconscious mind, where deeply rooted negative patterns are stored, to release everything that is not beneficial to the system and fully repair itself. We are moving through complex and stressful times; when we learn this transcendental healing method, we gain the capacity to truly heal ourselves, our loved ones, and everyone whom we encounter.

23

THE SPLENDOR OF NAAM YOGA

By revealing the hidden, essential truths of our various religious traditions and mystery systems, Naam Yoga allows us to begin to understand and relate to our Source, so that we may gain a greater understanding of ourselves. Indeed, the time has come for the Divine Spiritual Wisdom to be shared in the spirit and service of helping humankind. As Universal Kabbalists, we understand that we do not weaken our power by passing on the truth. To the contrary, we are strengthened, for the generous are blessed and sanctified through their acts.

Naam Yoga is a symbol of energy, and energy is the symbol of the magnetic field. Naam Yoga will turn you into a center of radiance and magnetic energy. It will give you a very cleansing and heart-opening effect and make you very beautiful. It will bestow upon you a luminous aura and give you the capacity to heal others with your presence, your touch and your words. Naam Yoga is the most powerful tool available for the removal of mental, physical and spiritual suffering. Naam Yoga leads to the development of a benevolent, magnetic personality and radiant spirit. By practicing Naam, you become revitalized with God's light and radiance. You begin to live from your heart instead of your head. Indeed, the scriptures tell us that so-called incurable illnesses vanish on the chords of a dedicated, consistent practice of Naam. By working with Naam, the body becomes attuned to a state of perfect healing, thereby granting you the love, faith and hope to sustain it. Conversely, when we neglect to vibrate Naam, our difficulties multiply. Become a student of the Divine Spiritual Wisdom and vibrate Naam so that you are open to the light of all worlds and realms, and are able to develop intuitive awareness, spiritual intelligence and health. Allow this spiritual technology to open your inner eye to the unseen and your inner ear to the unheard. Naam is the truth that leads to the great Truth. Truth is what guides us to happiness. Working with Naam Yoga is the path to indescribable ecstasy and the manifestation of your highest destiny and bliss. Naam Yoga allows you to receive wisdom, truth and love, or the source of purest knowledge, the principle of morality and the essential pure motive of will. Love and wisdom complete the spirit of truth, the inner light that illuminates the transcendental subjects within us. As each individual is infused with the kingdom of God, the kingdom of truth, morality and welfare, and the spirit of love, peace and light flourishes on a wide scale and leads to global healing. Naam Yoga accomplishes this by opening the organ that grants us a realization of higher truth. This organ is the intuitive sense faculty of the transcendental world. By practicing Naam, you eat the fruit of the Tree of Life, and it nourishes you with spiritual joy and healing.

Life is changing rapidly. We are at the advent of the Golden Age, which means that the planetary forces are at the cosmic steering wheel. We are engaged in a fierce battle between light and darkness as the zodiac signs use human beings as their vehicle for energetic war. The Earth is also engaged in combat. In order to survive and be free of misery, we must tap into the immortal, incorruptible principle within and develop it to the point that it devours the corruptible, mortal principle. The origin of man is God. The origin of the human race on earth is man's descent into matter. In most cases, human life is the manifestation of privation and struggle. However, at one time man occupied a much different place in the divine plan. We were once endowed with many superior faculties that made us a potent being, higher than the angels. Through misuse of free will, we descended from this first estate. Now, our individual and collective task is to become reintegrated into the archetype so that primitive Adam may be restored. Until this occurs, we will continue to suffer the consequences of the physical world. It is the yoga of Naam that can progressively restore our connection to the higher realms. By vibrating Naam and turning his spiritual eye upward in preparation for his return to his original home, man will revive his communication with, and rulership of, angelic beings. The pathway back to God is through a human body that vibrates Naam. We have been given a golden opportunity to reunite with God through this sacred practice.

Naam Yoga is the highest and most accessible form of yoga. Everyone, regardless of race, religion, age or physical condition, can practice it. When you are confronted with emotional or physical difficulties, when all support and hope has vanished, when you are under the power of obsessive sexual desire, anger and worldly attachments, when you have committed great sins and other mistakes, find relief in the practice of Naam Yoga. It will transport you away from darkness and into the bosom of the Divine, who is Eternal, Permanent and True. Naam will soothe your mind, body and soul. Vibrate the Naam, heal yourself, and help and uplift others.

*It is through the practice of the Word
that one merges with God,
because God is bound by the Word.*

CONCLUSION

Vibrate the Word and open your heart, and your inner being will be deeply imbued with the heavenly, protective color of the Love and Light of the Creator. Open your heart and vibrate the Word, and you will find the gate of salvation. Working with the Divine Spiritual Wisdom will make you calm and relaxed, happy and peaceful. These sacred teachings will quench your thirst for knowledge and open your heart, putting a smile upon your face and joy in your life. The Word is a simple, yet powerful science. In working with the Word, we partake of the Heavenly nourishment that gives radiant health and puts us on the path to fulfilling our destiny. Think for a moment how many people might benefit from these sacred teachings. Think of the joy, the comfort, the love, the faith and the hope that would blossom and grow in many hearts and souls by reconnecting them with the Divine Spiritual Wisdom. The happiness that these teachings inspire is the birthright of every living being. The Divine Spiritual Wisdom, Harmonyum healing, and the power of the Word can be used to fight life-threatening diseases. Indeed, a wide range of diseases, such as those with genetic roots and those that affect the blood and immune system, can be treated with the Divine Spiritual Wisdom, Harmonyum healing and the Word. Naam flows like a stream, the vibrations of which are guided and directed by conscious intelligences; for all the powers of nature are the expressions of the Word of God; all things are obeying the rhythmic law of the creative Word. Human beings are composed of the essences of all celestial planetary bodies; when we vibrate the Word and work with the Divine Spiritual Wisdom, this practice opens the heart and attracts the beneficial influences of the seven Creative Forces, or planetary bodies. The

Divine Spiritual Wisdom can cause man to rise above the seven Creative Forces of the Cosmos. These seven Forces govern all the kingdoms of the macrocosm and manifest in the twelve signs of the zodiac, which are represented by the human rib cage.

Practicing with the Word creates a stronger vibratory frequency within us, causing the lost inner organ to be activated. The opening of this spiritual faculty is the mystery of regeneration, of the vital union between God and man. This process of developing the inner faculty that allows us to receive God is our life's work. When the process is complete, the metaphysical and incorruptible principle rules over the terrestrial. Man begins to live, not in accordance with the principle of self-love, but in accordance with that of the Spirit and Truth for which he becomes a temple. We need the Word for total regeneration because it is not only the living symbol of the Sun, but also holds the inner and holy truth. Regeneration involves the sublimation of vice into virtue, and is the act of being reborn in the Spirit whereby the body and soul are penetrated by the heat of divine love and the light of divine intelligence that emanate from the divine fire held within self-consciousness and self-knowledge. In other words, when we tap into the divine fire of self-consciousness and self-knowledge, we receive and benefit from divine love and intelligence. Indeed, full regeneration cannot be attained without the action and vivifying touch of true love, for love is the creative force in both the individual and the divine. Naam will carry you across the poisonous ocean of worldly challenges with grace, and cause the God of incomparable beauty who fulfills our hopes and aspirations to sit in your heart. Both the chanter and listener are liberated, for they are drinking pure prana in the Lord's name. The essence of Naam is the practice of Truth. Vibrate the Naam and your tongue will be imbued with the Lord's Essence. Vibrate the Naam and your ten trillion cells will be imbued with the Love of the Lord. Vibrate the Naam and the radiant mark of purity will be written on your forehead. The Creator is pleased with those who vibrate the Word that enshrines their minds and hearts with the Sublime Essence of the Name of the Lord. Therefore, learn these sacred teachings, vibrate and drink in the sublime essence of the Naam, so that the Divinity of God may bless you, His piety warm you, and His love preserve you.

ABOUT THE AUTHOR

The work of Joseph Michael Levry, PhD, DD, MSIE, is an invitation to discover the intense and pure inner life of a brilliant mystic and Master teacher who, at the dawn of the 21st century, is bringing a renewal to spirituality. A tireless and dedicated teacher, writer, and lecturer, Dr. Levry, has traveled extensively throughout the United States, Europe and Asia for almost four decades. He travels nine months out of the year, teaching and lecturing in New York, Los Angeles, Sweden, Germany, Switzerland, Israel, the U.K., and France. By adopting such a rigorous travel schedule, Dr. Levry has been able to introduce many to the teachings of Divine Spiritual Wisdom as well as tune the frequency of the countries he visits to a higher level of vibration.

Dr. Levry, who is also known by his spiritual name Gurunam, has touched the lives of thousands of people of every race and religion guiding them through the process of self-healing and the realization of meaningful careers, healthy relationships and life-long dreams. Time and time again he has earned the trust of even the most skeptical through his precise diagnosis of physical ailments, and unique ability to see and analyze the energy field. He leads a Kabbalistic, research oriented life, imparting his knowledge without hesitation to all who wish to learn to improve life, restore health, and bring positive outcomes to the many problems of one's existence for a fulfilling and meaningful life.

Having experienced a high level of spiritual realization, God is a reality in his life. Dr. Levry places a strong emphasis on the fundamental oneness of all religions. He believes that Divine Spiritual Wisdom comes from one Source and although there are many paths to truth there is only One Supreme Way. Divine Spiritual Wisdom focuses on personal improvement and spiritual happiness which is the evidence of an authentic spiritual practice. In his books and lectures, he illuminates Kabbalistic teachings and symbols that were once kept secret within the doctrines of Judaism, Christianity, and other religions. These teachings are targeted to people of all faiths, as well as those with no specific faith. Although Dr. Levry does not focus on traditional religious requirements he promotes a Godly and conscientious lifestyle.

After 40 years of study, research, and teaching, Dr. Levry has created a unique synthesis of the powerful teachings of Universal Kabbalah and Naam Yoga® known as Divine Spiritual Wisdom. His training began at the age of 12 in the esoteric arts and sciences and he has been initiated into many spiritual orders, through which he learned the science of Kabbalah, Yoga, Asian energetic work, theology and today continues to learn from the limitless wisdom of God. Believing that nothing is done by chance, and that one can rewrite his or her destiny through the knowledge and application of this Divine Spiritual Wisdom, Dr. Levry is able to reach all who come to him with a willingness to actively initiate and participate in their own healing.

The men and women living and working with the disciplines of Divine Spiritual Wisdom have attuned themselves to the universal laws that flow in and throughout all of life, as well as the unseen powers and forces of nature. The combination of Universal Kabbalah and Naam Yoga produces the ultimate spiritual science, providing the necessary tools for healthy, effective living. This spiritual technology has shown individuals how to work in accordance with the laws of heaven and earth in order to achieve great success and contentment in their worldly experiences.

Many long time students of Divine Spiritual Wisdom have become both Naam Yogi and Universal Kabbalists. Together, they have formed an invisible empire of agents of light contributing to the positive evolution of humankind. Naam Yoga and the Universal Kabbalah contained within this vast science, is expanding quickly in America and abroad. This fast moving expansion is spurring the spread of many franchises in major metropolitan cities globally. There are extensive certification trainings, educational programs as well as the popularization of the powerful Naam music produced by Dr. Levry.

Fundamental to Divine Spiritual Wisdom is sacred music. Working with sacred music is akin to meditating on the divine truths that exist on a higher plane of reality. When we engage with sacred sounds, the depths of our being awaken fully to life. In practice, Universal Kabbalah is based on the proper use of the Word. In fact, the whole meditative life of the Universal Kabbalist is built upon the mystery of the Word. Universal Kabbalists believe in the power and efficacy of the Word which went forth at the creation of the world.

The Word is supreme. Since the fall of man, the power of God's Word has become our only hope for restoration. Dr. Levry teaches that by practicing with the Word humans can get to infinity without the necessity of interpretation or understanding from others. Devotees do not need to learn Hebrew in order to partake of the Divine Spiritual Wisdom. The emphasis is on the importance of seeing God in oneself, in others, and in every sacred teaching. Dr. Levry believes that to confine oneself to a particular belief system and deny all others puts us at risk of missing the vastness that is the knowledge of reality. In other words, much good eludes those who restrict themselves, for God is infinite, boundless, and too tremendous to be limited to one belief or another.

Dr. Levry established the Universal Force Healing Center in New York City. This amazing Center along with its Naam Yoga studio has healed and uplifted thousands of people during its 10 years of operation. In 2011, Naam Yoga LA opened in the Los Angeles county coastal city of Santa Monica, California. True to his vision, this is a new state of the art healing, research and Naam Yoga center dedicated to philanthropic activities that serve humankind. Naam Yoga LA is committed to intellectual and spiritual development as well as continuing and expanding its mission in the healing arts and sciences.

Naam Yoga LA is truly unique in the United States offering tools for maintaining and building a meaningful emotional and spiritual life along with attending to physical illnesses. These goals are accomplished several ways including sound and mudra therapy, yoga movement, meditation based on the purity of life, and the healing arts. In addition, Universal Force Inc. in conjunction with Naam Yoga LA is creating a research team devoted to natural and holistic healing with the purpose to diagnose and heal people from chronic cases of physical, emotional, and/or mental disturbance. Universal Force Healing Center operates according to the philosophy that spiritual diagnosis and treatment is of the utmost value and benefit. Its team includes highly qualified yogis and Kabbalists who are well versed in many diagnostic and healing procedures.

Dr. Levry is also the president of Rootlight, Inc., a publishing, production, and consulting company that produces sacred music and books that reflect the sacred teachings of Divine Spiritual Wisdom. In his various CDs and books he presents Universal Kabbalah as a way to know the unknown and see the unseen forces that govern our lives. He offers a wealth of Universal Kabbalah and Naam Yoga healing techniques, therapeutic exercises and meditations that allow one to strengthen the nervous system, balance the glandular system, renew the blood, merge with the higher worlds, and improve life. In addition, he has developed Harmonyum, a transcendental healing system born out of Universal Kabbalah. The "Harmonyum Healing System" activates the original seed and awakens the threefold soul, born of the threefold spirit, from the threefold body into self-consciousness and self-knowledge which brings about the balance and tranformation.

Dr. Levry maintains that the Divine Spiritual Wisdom contained in Universal Kabbalah creates within Man that which is known as *Mysterium Conjunctionis of the Alchemists,* symbolized by the Star of David that unites the upper heavenly triangle with the lower earthly triangle. This union of heaven and earth is the sacred miracle that causes the spirit to spiritualize matter, transforming our character, our personality, indeed our entire lives into pure spiritual gold.

Healing Beyond Medicine Series
by Dr. Joseph Michael Levry (Gurunam)

BOOKS:

Alchemy of Love Relationships
A practical guide to creating successful relationships through the application of spiritual principles from Universal Kabbalah and Naam Yoga®. The application of these principles will completely change your approach to life and relationships. This is an invaluable book for a richer and more fulfilling love relationship. *Also available in Spanish.*

Lifting the Veil: The Divine Code
This book allows you to penetrate the high mysteries of the Kabbalah by presenting this timeless wisdom in a practical, workable and understandable way. In this book, you will find a time-proven formula to experience a life of grace and joy. Included are over 50 meditations and simple exercises to enhance your health, balance the mind, body and spirit, and develop intuition. *Also available in German and Spanish.*

The Code of the Masters: Universal Kabbalah with Naam Yoga®
You will also learn how Master yogis and Kabbalists use their hands, along with the mantric science, to connect with the heavens for healing and happiness. Practicing the science of Naam will strengthen the vibratory frequency within you, opening your heart and activating the soul. This book reveals the spiritual truth regarding the Fall and Nature of Man, Kabbalistic Palmistry, Naam Yoga and the present state of our world. Learning these sacred and timeless teachings will put hope in our souls, faith in our spirits, and love in our hearts, and from that place we are able to see the beauty and light of life.

The Divine Doctor: Healing Beyond Medicine
This book gives you the key to numerous mysteries in medicine and healing which are completely unknown within ordinary medical practices, thereby giving you access to timeless healing technologies that are the birthright of humankind. *The Divine Doctor* reveals the precise methods for working with the spiritual body to achieve self-healing and maintain vibrant health. It will also guide you through these techniques, so that you may recover more quickly from illness and become healthy. *The Divine Doctor* is for all yogis, Kabbalists, doctors, serious health practitioners and anyone who desires to achieve self-healing and help others heal through the application of profound meditations and practical techniques.

The Healing Fire of Heaven: Mastering the Invisible Sunlight Fluid for Healing and Spiritual Growth (Previously titled The Splendor of the Sun)
This book will show you practical ways of connecting with the sun in order to capture its many benefits and blessings. Working with the sun is one of the highest, most potent and effective spiritual systems you can come across on this earth. Working with the sun will cause your soul to become active and your spiritual powers to become operative, showing clear visible signs in your mind, spirit and physical body.

ADVANCED SELF-STUDY COURSE (LEVELS 1–4)
The Sacred Teachings of Kabbalah and Naam Yoga®
Kabbalah and Naam Yoga® are two ancient and powerful sciences for spiritual growth, and for understanding one's self in relation to the Universe. This course is a compelling and extremely practical masterpiece of Universal Kabbalah. The sacred teachings of Kabbalah have been presented in a practical, do-able and understandable way. You will be given some of the most effective meditations and prayers that Kabbalah and Naam Yoga® have to offer. The essence of Kabbalah, that was previously hidden and confusingly presented in various books, has been decoded and put into a form that is effective and powerful in its application. By working with this course, all the dormant qualities and virtues in you are brought to full life, resulting in improved health and well-being on all levels.

DVD:
Radiant Health with Naam Yoga®: *A Dynamic Meditation Practice in Seated Pose*
This DVD contains two complete Naam Yoga meditation sequences for balancing complex disease, strengthening the heart and improving well being. This practice is a cellular infiltration of the solar force causing every atom of your being to scintillate with light and life allowing for vital regeneration of the entire body. Excellent for daily practice. Contains a useful mudra reference.

SACRED MUSIC SERIES CDS:
Blissful Spirit — Har Gobinday/Ganpati Mantra/Wahe Guru/Ong
These sound vibrations eliminate mental impurities and cause the spirit to blossom, while bestowing divine grace and radiance.

Green House — *Har Gobinday (II) / Har Haray Haree Wahe Guru (III) / Ad Such / Calm Heart*
These sound vibrations extend the power of projection and protection in the personality. They help open the door to opportunities and attract blessings.

Healing Beat of Naam — *Healing Musical Energies*
The sound vibrations on this CD are powerful spiritual seeds. When planted in a person's heart, they will sprout the most beautiful healing tree that will, in turn, bear delicious, sweet fruit. This CD features vocals ascending the musical scale to amplify the healing processes of the body.

Healing Fire — *Ong / Prayer of Light / 12 Seed Sounds*
These sound vibrations give youth, beauty and spiritual illumination. They work on the glandular system and organs. A regular practice of listening to this CD or chanting along with it promotes good health and helps develop intuitive intelligence.

Heaven's Touch — *Guru Ram Das / Sat Narayan / Mystical Ivory Coast*
These sound vibrations bring grace, blessings and internal peace. The sound current on the first track synchronizes your energy and expands the aura. It is also for emergency saving grace and spiritual guiding light. The second sound current cleanses the emotions, creates internal peace and allows you to project outer peace. The third track moves you into a meditative space with rhythm.

House of Ram — *Shri Ram Jai Ram / Harmonic Ram / Kabbalistic Om*
For nourishing and healing the Aura: RAM activates the purifying fire within, burning away every negative vibration from our physical, mental and spiritual bodies. Ram is the mantra of miracles that will remove the barriers between you and your higher self. It attracts the creativity and blessings of the entire Universe and beckons them to rush to your aid, elevating and uplifting every area of your life that is in need of energy. The mantra found on the first track brings joy and happiness on the spot. It is said that those who vibrate it find complete fulfillment in their life.

Invocation of Divine Light — *Connection & Guidance*
The sound vibrations on this CD are powerful prayers to invoke the light and to open the connection between the self and the Divine for guidance and Light. They help us break through blocks and release negative patterns. You will become a magnet for the beneficent forces of the universe.

Kabbalah for Healing — *Opening the Heart & Bringing Healing*
The combination of these ancient and sacred Hebrew words of power are designed to open the heart and bring healing. By working with these sound vibrations you will merge with the Creator, realize the greater, loving omnipresence and power that is God. You will be reminded of where you came from, why you are here, where you will return to, and of your true destiny. With this awareness, you can become a pure channel of love, peace, and light to all, and your life will be full of grace and blessings.

Lumen de Lumine — *For Opening the Heart and Touching the Soul*
This sound vibration surrounds those who chant or listen to it with a blanket of light. Just listen to it and it will purify and strengthen your aura. Play it in a room and it will clear the energy in a short time. Go to sleep with it and you will wake up revitalized. When faced with challenges, play it continuously; it will eat the darkness out of your life.

Mystic Light — *RaMa Ram Ram/Hallelu-ya/Lumen De Lumine (II)/ Har Haray Haree/Sophia*
The sound vibrations on Mystic Light revitalize the energy flow within the body and make the aura strong, bright and beautiful. They not only affect the two brain hemispheres and bring you into balance, but they also draw down the protective light and grace of heaven. They give you light, healing, and strength.

Naam Groove-The Essential Remix — *I Am, Love Peace Light/Ong Namo/ The Journey (NEW! Instrumental)/Ajai Alai/Sat Nam Har Haree*
It's time to get your Naam groove on! Bringing together fun and uplifting melodies and infusing them into long-time favorites, *The Naam Groove* will breathe new life into your yoga, meditation or healing practice as it creates a fun and upbeat atmosphere everywhere it's played. Enjoy these heart-opening combinations of sacred words and healing rhythms while commuting, working, cooking, working out and studying. These tracks have been especially remixed to magnify their healing effects on the psyche and nervous system.

Naam Lounge— *Balancing Instrumental Beats*
The music and rhythmic beats on this CD possess strong healing qualities and are very uplifting. Working with this CD will create a connection between you and your soul. This form of communion is like a sweet spiritual wine. If you work constantly with these healing rhythms, you will find

www.rootlight.com

that they bring order and balance to your life; everything within you will become ideally structured and harmonious.

OM House — *Activating the Primal Force Within*
The sacred sound OM/AUM on Om House is mystically vibrated in the most potent and correct way—ONG/AUNG—in order to heal, empower and rejuvenate the chanter or listener. It creates the healing space. This sound is thought to have special universal powers for the creation of worldly things. The divine word OM, which is nothing more than AUM, is pregnant with mysterious power. OM stimulates the psychic centers, and is known to have certain therapeutic value.

Pure Naam — *Gobinday Har Har Har Har/Har Haray Haree–Wahe Guru/Wahe Guru Wahe Jio/Guru Ram Das (Remix)*
These powerful sound vibrations cause your projection to cut through all negativity in your daily life. They bestow courage, willpower and confidence. The special combination of voice and melody on the second track will surround you with an aura of prosperity and protection. These sacred words of power act as a healing balm for the mind and emotions that resolves and eliminates all ego problems and mental diseases while positively stimulating your nervous, glandular and digestive systems.

Ra Ma Da Sa — *To heal and/or maintain balance and health (ORIGINAL)*
This sound vibration cuts across time and space and brings healing. It maintains, strengthens and improves your health. It can generate beneficial energy in hospital rooms and places of recovery. It will also create a peaceful and productive environment in the workplace. Families can benefit from its harmonizing effects on the home, children and even pets. (Set to the healing tune of Pachabel's Cannon.) See also *The Healing Spirit of Ra Ma Da Sa*.

Soul Trance — *Wahe Guru (II)/Har/Love, Peace, Light to All (SaReGaMa)*
These sound vibrations help awaken the soul, so you may manifest your higher destiny. They help give clarity, stability, and harmony. For depression and mental imbalances

Sounds of the Ether — *Ad Such/I AM/Aim/Hari Har/The Fire of Prayer*
The sound vibrations on this CD open the door to opportunity, good fortune and the realization of one's dreams and ambitions. When you chant and/or listen to them, you are calling upon the divine helping hand to assist you in attracting true happiness. As a result, you will be blessed with a fulfilling and successful earthly life.

The Flow of Naam — *Mul Mantra/Guru Gaitri Mantra/Sat Nam Wahe Guru/Love, Peace and Light*
Vibrating the sacred sound current, or Naam, will turn you into a center of radiance and magnetic energy. It will bestow upon you a beautiful, luminous aura and give you the capacity to heal others with your presence, touch and words. Naam is the most powerful tool available for opening the heart and for the removal of mental, physical and spiritual suffering. By vibrating Naam, you are able to develop intuitive awareness, spiritual intelligence and health.

The Healing Spirit of Ra Ma Da Sa — *To Heal and/or Maintain Balance and Health*
(See Ra Ma Da Sa description. This is set to three different melodies.)

The Seal of Higher Destiny — *Eck Ong Kar Sat Nam Siri Wahe Guru*
This is a Naam that projects the mind beyond the realm of everyday earthly consciousness into the infinity of the cosmos and awakens the soul to one's higher destiny. It brightens your energy, wipes out karma, and increases your sense of personal relatedness to the infinite identity.

Touch of Naam — *Developing the Power of Speech*
The sound vibrations on this CD greatly amplify one's ability to manifest the things they want in this life. When practiced with reverence, these sacred words of power will elevate the self into the bosom of the Divine and establish a direct link with the Spirit.

Triple Mantra — *For Protection and to Clear Obstacles*
This sound vibration clears all types of psychic and physical obstacles in one's daily life. It will strengthen your magnetic field and keep negativity away, and it is a powerful protection against car, plane or other accidents. This mantra cuts through all opposing vibrations, thoughts, words and actions.

For more information on Harmonyum® Healing, Naam Yoga®, Universal Kabbalah®, Special Events, new sacred music releases, personal reports through the *Akashic Record*, and to receive our free *Light of Insight* e-newsletter please visit our website: **www.rootlight.com**

Order Form

Title	Each	Qty.	Subtotal
BOOKS			
Alchemy of Love Relationships	$25	x ____ =	____
Alchemy of Love Relationships (SPANISH)	$28	x ____ =	____
Lifting the Veil	$23	x ____ =	____
The Code of the Masters	$28	x ____ =	____
The Divine Doctor	$25	x ____ =	____
The Healing Fire of Heaven	$23	x ____ =	____
ADVANCED SELF-STUDY COURSE			
Level 1	$360	x ____ =	____
Level 2	$360	x ____ =	____
Level 3	$360	x ____ =	____
Level 4	$360	x ____ =	____
DVD			
Radiant Health with Naam Yoga	$30	x ____ =	____
CDS			
Blissful Spirit	$19	x ____ =	____
Green House	$19	x ____ =	____
Healing Fire	$19	x ____ =	____
Heaven's Touch	$19	x ____ =	____
Healing Beat of Naam	$19	x ____ =	____
House of Ram *(new 2011!)*	$19	x ____ =	____
Invocation of Divine Light	$19	x ____ =	____
Kabbalah for Healing	$19	x ____ =	____
Lumen de Lumine	$19	x ____ =	____
Mystic Light	$19	x ____ =	____
OM House	$19	x ____ =	____
Naam Groove *(new 2011!)*	$19	x ____ =	____
Naam Lounge	$19	x ____ =	____
Pure Naam *(new 2011!)*	$19	x ____ =	____
Ra Ma Da Sa *(Original Version)*	$19	x ____ =	____
Soul Trance	$19	x ____ =	____
Sounds of the Ether	$19	x ____ =	____
The Flow of Naam	$19	x ____ =	____
The Healing Spirit of Ra Ma Da Sa	$19	x ____ =	____
The Seal of Higher Destiny	$19	x ____ =	____
Touch of Naam	$19	x ____ =	____
Triple Mantra	$19	x ____ =	____

SUBTOTAL _____

Shipping & Handling _____

N.Y. residents add 8.65% sales tax _____

TOTAL DUE _____

Shipping in USA: add $5.50 for 1st item, $.50 each additional item.

Prices subject to change (8/11). Allow up to two weeks for shipping for Self-Study Courses

PLEASE CONTINUE ORDER ON OTHER SIDE OF FORM>>>

PAYMENT INFORMATION:
(Please print clearly)

Payment enclosed: ❏ Check   ❏ Money Order
Please make checks payable to: **Rootlight, Inc.**

Please charge order to my credit card: ❏ Visa   ❏ Mastercard

NAME AS SHOWN ON CARD:

CREDIT CARD NUMBER

EXPIRATION DATE MM/DD/YYYY

SIGNATURE

BILLING ADDRESS *(if different from shipping)*:

ADDRESS

CITY   STATE   ZIP

PHONE (if we have questions about your order)

SHIPPING INFORMATION:

NAME

ADDRESS

CITY   STATE   ZIP

PHONE (if we have questions about your order)

E-MAIL

Thank you for your order!

ROOTLIGHT, INC.
15 Park Avenue Suite 7C, New York, NY 10016
TOLL FREE IN U.S.: (888) 852-2100   INTERNATIONAL: (212) 769-8115
FAX: (805) 384-9091   EMAIL: orders@rootlight.com
Please visit us at www.rootlight.com